MENTAL HEALTH DISABILITY

Perception vs. Reality

By

Louis Bianco, RN, CPS

Mental Health DisABILITY: Perception vs. Reality

by Louis Bianco, RN, CPS

Published by Grace & Hope Consulting, LLC

P.O. Box 104 - Dillsburg, PA 17019

www.graceandhopeconsulting.com

Editor: Catherine Hughes

Cover Artist: Bianca Correll

ASIN: B087B43T6T

ISBN: 9798638911331

"Information on Wellness should not be reserved solely for those in crisis to help them out of it. It should be shared with the healthy in hopes of avoiding crisis altogether."

-Louis Bianco

Table of Contents

PROLOGUE

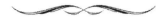

My name is Louis Bianco. I am a Registered Nurse and a Certified Peer Support Specialist. I have had my share of struggles and difficulties in regard to mental illness, and I have also worked professionally with others going through similar struggles. I have worked with all ages, races, and genders. I have seen the rich and the poor in the same room, desperately trying to put the pieces of their broken lives back together. As a professional, I have been in family meetings with supportive loved ones and family meetings with relatives that never showed up.

There are many misconceptions about the criteria necessary to actually have a diagnosed mental illness. Simply put, if one's emotional or mental stress prohibits them from performing their "normal" level of functioning, they may be mentally ill, or that is how it was presented to me throughout my years in the field. Consequently, there are many theories about what causes someone to lose their ability to function. Although we have slight understandings of subjects such as chemical imbalances and faulty cognition, one thing for me remains true. Mental illness is confusing and can be debilitating.

Personally, I believe in the "nature and nurture" theory. I believe that people can have genetic dispositions that leave them vulnerable to our current understandings of what mental illness is. Hereditary mental illness has been researched and proven. Although I disagree with certain items regarding the definitive nature in which we discuss this concept, I have never been one to argue with facts.

However, the ways in which a person is raised and conditioned shapes who they become, especially at younger ages. So if a parent suffers from something emotional or cognitive in nature and exhibits the behaviors that are associated with any specific mental

2

illness, the child being raised by them is exposed to it the day they are born.

Generation after generation demonstrates the same dysfunction. It surely appears genetic, but the idea that years of exposure doesn't have something to do with the child becoming ill, is foolish in my opinion. This could mean that mental illness can be as contagious as it is genetic, in a sense. The argument to the previously stated hypothesis exists within families where only one of many children end up unable to function.

Same parents, same rules, similar genetics.

This is where trauma comes in.

Any type of trauma experienced in one's life can become the accelerator of symptoms that already exist or even wake up dormant afflictions. This trauma, or perceived trauma, acts as the catalyst that ultimately opens "Pandora's Box," or that genetic disposition to mental illness and all of the symptoms that come with it. Such is the case with the young man whose case study I would like to share with you.

3

I'll admit, I often question the professionalism of what I have decided to do, but I have never been able to forget his unique journey. This is a person, who even at a very young age, motivated me to work harder at my job and in my life. He is someone who continually took beatings, although physical abuse was never a concern in his life. These beatings were from life, both self-inflicted and incurred from the innocent ignorance of those around him trying to "help."

This is not to say that he was perfect, quite the opposite really. He made plenty of mistakes and deserved to be disliked by some of those whose path he crossed. He wasn't always the most compassionate person. He was extremely selfish at times. But even in the face of mistakes or failures, he trudged along. He admitted fault, he apologized, and he tried harder after every roadblock. Sure, he also complained, had pity parties and emotionally manipulated those around him during periods of weakness.

Living with his brain could not have been easy. But as he got older, I found myself wondering if he was truly ill, or just misunderstood. He showed us as many talents as

4

he did symptoms. His resiliency and his ability to improve upon designated weaknesses were a testament to his intelligence and courage. Constantly creating new and better versions of himself showed me his work ethic and durability.

So here I am, writing this story, complete with documentation from our sessions together and other documents written by his hand.

I am not a trained writer. I know very little about formatting or how to "appropriately" create a story. But this story must be told, and I know enough about this case, and the field of mental health itself, to be qualified to tell it.

My intention is to raise questions about the system itself.

I will be giving you, the reader, a complete background of his life and the circumstances that led to a court ruling of "disabled" in his young adulthood. Yes, he was deemed disabled in the eyes of the state following an inability to function in society. Was this because he was truly mentally ill, or because he adhered to the

5

warnings and guidelines drilled into his head following a breakdown in his teenage years? Did he have an illness that made him disabled, or was he the product of a greater dysfunction - social disability?

It is not my intention to point fingers.

All members of his family, and treatment team, had the best of intentions, as did he. His life was never absent of love; instead, it was at times misguided by a much more prevalent and powerful fear - a fear that was as instrumental in his survival as it was in his demise. It was a fear experienced by himself, and the adults around him. The more someone cared for him, the more fearful they were, and the more they acted out of fear. Were the decisions made by the adults in his life done to protect him or to protect the adults from their own discomforts and lack of understanding?

It is important to me that I reiterate my intentions. I do not want to blame anyone.

I was as much a part of his care as anyone during his formative years. The same years in which he experienced the worst of his condition. We all tried, including him. He

6

wasn't usually oppositional when treatment was concerned. Frustrated? Certainly, but when we told him he needed a certain medication, he took it. When we told him something was a symptom, he paid attention, whether we thought he did or not.

His family listened to us (the medical professionals) attentively. Everyone involved was on board. We were going to figure this out and fix it. Although we saw periods of what we believed were recovery, he ended up with nothing by age 34. He was a 34 year old, attractive, fit, intelligent, sensitive and caring adult male, now immobile. He was a Registered Nurse and Certified Peer Support Specialist, unemployed. He was a creative, compassionate, well-spoken human being with a spirit that had been slowly dying for 20 years. Although not absent of faults, he was a good man. He was also broke, living with his parents, and officially disabled. How? Let's find out, shall we?

Chapter 1: A Gift and A Curse

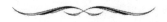

I'll never forget the first time I met him. He was seven years old. He had large glasses on and a patch over his left eye in order to strengthen his vision on the right side.

Documentation from his internist showed that he was small for his age in both height and weight, although his head was actually measured to be quite large for his frame. He was every bit as precocious as his teachers had described and demonstrated excellent communication skills during his standardized intelligence test. We tested everyone at this age and it appeared, based on our initial

8

assessment, that a follow up would be necessary as he continued to mature. The student was polite and maintained eye contact throughout our initial interaction. He was a very pleasant child, and I enjoyed his ability to hold a conversation. He had a charisma and kindness about him that was hard to find in anyone, let alone a child.

Unfortunately, this wasn't the only time I met with him, and our following meeting, merely months later, had nothing to do with our findings from his intelligence test. I remembered that he had been described by his teachers and family as sensitive, hypersensitive at times, becoming overly upset while having difficulty understanding basic concepts such as right and wrong or fairness.

I feared that these descriptions from my peers may have clouded my vision when he arrived at my office holding back his tears, while clenching his mother's hand. It was then that his mother told me he had been complaining about one of his classmates touching him inappropriately while talking about sexually explicit material. It was obvious to me that neither the child or his mother had any idea how to handle the situation.

He proceeded to explain to me everything that happened, reciting exactly what was said to him during this experience. It was clear, as I watched his eye contact fade and his posture slouch, that he was traumatized. Unfortunately, for this child and his family, situations such as this one were not talked about as openly in the early 90's as they are now. The majority of the adults associated with this situation felt it was best to try and minimize its gravity. We instructed him to avoid this specific classmate at all costs, but ultimately kept him in class with his perpetrator and required minimal follow up. No punishment was enforced and the two children continued to learn in the same classroom for the remainder of the year.

As I look back, I regret assuming that this child was overreacting and just demonstrating what was previously assessed as hypersensitivity. I remember initially thinking to myself that old cliché: "kids will be kids." I often wonder, had I realized the damage that this initial trauma would cause my dear friend later in life, if

I could have done more as a professional. Knowing what we know now, over 20 years later, I realize that this was just one of the many oversights that occurred during the care for this young man.

Here is the documentation from the meeting in which he and his mother reported the violation to me. Please remember that at this time, such events were not thought to be traumatic, especially given the fact that both parties involved were very young. We have since learned much more about the negative effects such experiences can create.

October 21st, 1990 @ 0800

Student is a seven year old Caucasian male. Student and mother entered my office hand in hand. Student was observed as distraught, with poor eye contact (looking at ground) and slumped posture. Initial assessment showed that student was alert and oriented x3, but presented with a broad affect. Student needed prompting to give answers to very basic questions regarding name and date. Compared to previous interactions, student's communication was basically nonexistent, often retreating into his mother's arms instead of conversing. Mother

11

stated that student had been complaining about a peer touching him inappropriately in his genital region. Upon further investigation, consumer stated the name of the accused, as well as what was said during the interaction. Student stated that his peer was discussing the physical appearance of his step mother, mainly her breasts, and verbalizing that this made said peer aroused. Peer then asked the student if he was aroused as well and rubbed student's genitals with his hands. The children were apparently on a bus heading to their required swimming class with the rest of their grade. Student did not tell his teacher when it initially occurred and instead told mother upon arriving home after school. Mother states that student was tearful throughout the evening, sobbing and verbalizing a discomfort going back to school the next day. Mother then stated that student continued to verbalize discomfort in the morning and required her to drive him to school as he was unable to get on the bus. After discussing the incidents with both the student and his mother, it has been decided that the school staff will be made aware of the situation; however, no punishment will be issued at this time. Upon my recommendation, the student is not to go anywhere near said peer during school hours. This includes recess, lunch periods, bus rides, etc. It was also suggested that the teacher change seats around in the classroom

12

to ensure a safe and appropriate distance between the two children. Although student is tearful and reserved, it is my assessment that nothing further needs to be done at this time. Based on previous descriptions of student's emotional lability when dealing with difficult situations, current behaviors are assessed as age appropriate for specific child. Both student and mother agree to said terms at this time. Staff was notified. Will follow up with teacher to make sure all interventions are implemented.

Louis Bianco RN, CPS - end of visit note.

Although the situation was quite intense, the young man and his family recovered from the incident and continued on. As I stated previously, I knew following his initial intelligence testing that this young man may indeed be gifted. He continued to mature both intellectually and emotionally, and it was decided that further intelligence testing was required. It was decided that a more specific IQ test was necessary and I once again found myself interacting with this gregarious young man.

He appeared to be back to his normal self following the trauma he suffered the previous year. His overall affect was bright during our interaction, showing no signs of the previously mentioned sensitivity, although the setting was very low stress and the instructions were direct. I simply had him perform a series of tests that assessed his ability to problem solve and think critically. He appeared to have little difficulty with any of the tests and remained calm throughout the entirety of the process.

Per his mother, I did not divulge his exact IQ to him, and I will continue to honor her request, at this time, by maintaining confidentiality in this matter. Needless to say, I was right. He was gifted, based on how we defined it 20 years ago. We placed him in the gifted program at his elementary school, referred to as "Special Interest." He excelled almost immediately in said program, showing high levels of creative thinking and even winning local competitions involving others in similar classes at neighboring schools.

His ability to interact with his peers and adults was quite impressive, showing an almost effortless charisma.

I felt confident that we handled the previous situation appropriately, and it appeared that there were no long term effects from his incident. He was excelling academically, athletically, and socially. He had little difficulty making friends and continued to demonstrate communication skills beyond his age. He was once again demonstrating his pleasant disposition, and it looked like the most difficult of times were behind him.

August 30th, 1991 @ 1330

Student is an eight year old Caucasian male. Referred by educational staff in regard to IQ and possible placement in gifted programs. Received permission from student's mother to do standard IQ testing on the school premises. Student presented as alert and oriented x3 with a bright affect. Student was not on any psychotropic medications and was described as well adjusted in classroom setting and at home. Interactions at time of assessment showed this to be accurate. Referral did note that student was prone to crying spells often during interactions with siblings and peers, but nothing outside of what is considered age appropriate. Issued IQ test. Student showed little difficulty during assessment and remained pleasant throughout the process. Able to follow instructions

15

with little difficulty. Upon receiving test results it is my recommendation that consumer be enrolled in gifted program at elementary school. Parents and teachers were notified of results. Mother requested that the results not be discussed with student. Individual Education Program (IEP) will be implemented at the start of the Special Interest program and will be repeated annually by classroom staff.

Louis Bianco RN, CPS - end of visit note.

Chapter 2: Warning Signs

It was quite some time until I saw him again. Periodically, throughout his time in elementary school, he would show up with his mother after having difficulty getting his day started. From time to time, they would appear at my door exasperated from what seemed to be another tiresome argument over attending class. He was never mean to me, but it was clear that he was giving his mother a run for her money. I remember how tired she looked, but she never wavered in her endless pursuit to figure out what was going on. We rarely talked about the initial incident that brought him to my office, seemingly never putting two and two together so to speak. It was as if the trauma he experienced was a thing of the past and in no way could have caused these outbreaks.

He followed our lead most of the time. I could see the gears in his head constantly turning and, although he rarely spoke out against any of my directives, there were times that I knew he was confused and possibly disagreed with my judgment. He continued to flourish, even under these circumstances, and we all assumed that he was just sensitive. We (the adults in his life) believed that he just needed thicker skin, he just needed to toughen up. He participated in school activities and took a liking to music early on in his life, playing the clarinet and singing in the choir. I remember that he loved to draw as well. It was not until 1995 that we once again crossed paths.

It was the summer before his first day of sixth grade. In his school district, multiple elementary schools converged into one of two middle schools, and those two middle schools then all attended the same high school. He had completed elementary school with ease, at least as far as academics were concerned. He maintained solid friendships and participated in all of the associated activities involved with childhood: sleepovers, birthday parties, organized sports, etc. He continued to grow into himself, still small in stature, but with a personality that was as large as anyone I had ever worked with previously. I will never forget his ability to make me laugh out loud even though I was much older than he was. In my profession, it is important to maintain healthy distance from those that you interact with once they are able to get back on their feet. I often thought about how he was doing, not because I was worried about him, but because I truly believed that he was destined for something wonderful. It never crossed my mind, all of those years back, that he would ever suffer from lingering effects of that one fateful day. In all honesty, I didn't even think that there was any connection when he was once again referred to me for a meeting.

It appeared, based on the information I received prior to our appointment, that he was possibly struggling with his self esteem. He continued to love competition. It was stated in his referral that he occasionally would become tearful when his soccer team would lose, but it never stopped him from attending practices and putting forth maximum effort in all of his contests and practices. He

19

had difficulty being taken out of the games and replaced with people who didn't practice as hard as he did or have the same skill set he had. He was growing up in an age in which we, as a society, were realizing that everyone deserves a chance. Unfortunately, in our foolishness, we began denying people with natural talent those same opportunities in order to make others feel more confident. By making sure we improved the self esteem of the less talented, we were actually decreasing the self esteem of the more talented. Our belief in the idea of "no child left behind" backfired, as we were oblivious to the fact that we were decreasing his confidence in order to improve others. I digress.

He and his twin brother had taken a liking to basketball at this time as well, and were attending a basketball camp on the campus of his future high school. This was his first time getting to meet and interact with peers that would soon be his classmates in his new school setting. Interactions like this were slightly threatening to him. It often took him a little bit of time to adjust to any new situation, and this was no different. Adding to the previously described stress was what seemed to be a high demand that he put on himself to excel. He had no formal experience in basketball, just the lessons he received from his brother in law, on the street, at the front of his family's home.

The first few days of the camp were described as somewhat taxing for him. He appeared to get down on himself for not being as good of a player as many of his peers. I remember him telling me about free throw drills, in which they would put the campers in groups of six and have each one shoot ten free throws individually in front of the other group members. He usually made the least, keeping track of his percentage along with everyone else in his group. It was not easy for him to just enjoy something. It was not easy for him to understand that he couldn't just be good at something immediately. In fact, after talking with him about the whole experience, it very well may have been quite difficult.

I wish, for his sake, that lackluster basketball skills were the only obstacle he was faced with at this specific camp. Unfortunately, this just wasn't the case, and I soon learned about the incident that sent him over the edge emotionally. He was becoming more comfortable with

21

the other boys at his camp. They were often put into five on five competitions and he was able to utilize the few skills he possessed more under these parameters. Following one of the games, at the end of the camp session, he was observed by his peers putting his arm around one of his teammates to say, "Good game!" One of the other kids who saw this decided to make fun of him. This was a kid he had actually known about prior to the camp.

This kid was a very good basketball player.

This kid was very popular.

This kid called him "gay."

As we talked more about his recollection of the incident, I saw that he was once again becoming tearful. I immediately recalled all of the previous information I have read about his sensitivity. I again assumed, at this time, that he was showing weakness and that he needed to figure out a way to get over it. Part of me believed this advice to be true. I tried to explain to him that people are always going to try to hurt our feelings and that we cannot give up on what we enjoy because of what others

22

say. I'm sure I used phrases like "no big deal" and "relax" during our discussion. I'm not sure, at that time, that I realized how upset this actually made him. Again, this was close to 20 years ago.

Homosexuality was not discussed and carried a much greater stigma than it does now, mainly because we, as a society, were ignorant about it. It was used as an insult at this time, and, based on his reaction, it was perceived that way as well. We continued to talk for the rest of our hour session. I had him do deep breathing exercises so that he was able to speak clearly. We really tried to focus on what exactly it was that made him so upset.

This was the first time I noticed that he began to say, "I don't know" to my questions.

He had always been so eloquent when he spoke, and I will never forget when he started to shift to a more dismissive approach. He obviously wasn't pleased with the direction our conversation had gone, and although he remained polite throughout, I knew he was holding back anger.

That's the thing about this kid. I believe he had a rage inside of him that even he was afraid to unleash for fear of what he was actually capable of doing. I believe this rage became so intense at times that the only way he was able to experience any type of safe release from this energy was to cry. He told me he cried the day this happened too, which didn't help him in the moment. Being emotional was just more fuel for the other kids to hop on the bandwagon and engage in their early onset homophobia. I asked him towards the end of our session, briefly, about whether or not there was any truth to the comments the others had made. I wanted him to know there he was safe to disclose any feelings he had and also that he would be accepted regardless of his sexual preference. He told me about his girlfriend at the time and verbalized no romantic interest or attraction to those of the same sex. However, this didn't appear to be enough clarification for him, as he was more concerned with what others thought and were possibly saying than what he knew to be true.

After he left that day, I remember thinking to myself that I had really screwed up this time. I felt like he was

24

possibly worse off leaving than he was coming in. He had requested that I not share all of this with his parents and I honored his wishes. He was almost a teenager at this point and I felt that he didn't need to share every incident he experienced with his mother and father. There were times, as you will see moving ahead, that I had no choice but to share our discussions with the adults in his life, but I didn't believe this was one of them.

July 8th, 1995 @0900

Student is now twelve years of age. Student is currently not on any psychotropic medications and has no mental health diagnoses. Alert and oriented x3. Referred to me following an incident involving several peers at a basketball camp. Presented with a flat affect, although able to show emotion during periods of sadness. Poor eye contact. Slumped posture with head in hands often during interaction. Tearful with periods of crying during discussion. Denies any suicidal or homicidal ideation. Following initial assessment, student was asked about specific incident. Verbalized that he had put his arm around a peer and was then called "gay" by others. Student states that he began to cry once his peers began calling him names, and states that the teasing became worse following this. Student verbalized not

25

wanting to continue to attend camp and said, "I didn't even want to go in the first place." Processed situation with student and tried to help clarify understanding of self. Student stated, "I have a girlfriend, and I don't understand why they would call me that. Most of them go to school with her." Tried to redirect student back to self understanding and self worth, but student was observed as preoccupied with what others had said and were possibly thinking. Attempted to help student put situation in perspective with little success. Student was then observed as having closed body language and began saying, "I don't know" to all questions asked. Observed student tapping left foot with labored breathing as if frustrated. Educated student on de-escalation techniques. Student verbalized one technique that he found helpful following instruction: deep breathing. Discussed with student the importance of trying to practice this specific technique during periods of extreme stress. Student acknowledged instructions and agreed non-verbally to continue to practice said technique prior to leaving session. Asked Student once more if there was anything else we needed to discuss at which point Student shook head signifying a "no" response. Affect remained unchanged upon student exiting. Left under care of mother.

Louis Bianco RN, CPS - end of visit note.

Chapter 3: The Calm

He had a successful middle school career. I had heard that he ran into some difficulty in the beginning of his sixth grade year because he ended up in the same homeroom as the kid who made fun of him at camp. It seems that the bullying continued on for a bit but he was able to maintain a clear head and rise above it. I always admired his desire to not be a victim regardless of the circumstances he found himself in. He would sulk and complain, explaining why something wasn't fair or right. He would ask why others did what they did. I always felt helpless as if he was asking me for answers I couldn't give him. I rarely had answers for him. However, when push came to shove, he never wished harm on others, although

I am sure he may have hoped they would experience something that humbled them. Something humiliating that gave them an empathy they currently did not possess. I did not see this as evil or vengeful, he was just a child after all - a bright, conflicted child.

For the most part, he took a lot on the chin and then passionately discussed it at home, emoting intensely and misdirecting his frustration on those he trusted, especially his mother. He needed to dump it all off somewhere because he knew more was coming. This was the only way he could keep up this act he created. His sense of humor and personality in general helped him gain the popularity he dreamt of and he even became friends with the person who previously hurt his feelings. He seemed to believe that none of his friends would like the real him, so he paraded around in his "class clown" costume. He wanted so badly to be accepted. He remained in the band and reached the first chair in the clarinet. He joined the choir, as well as taking art classes. He even won a high school poetry contest in the category he entered and took second in the overall competition. His teacher encouraged him to continue to write. He had

29

such a passion for the arts and even made his way onto the stage in his school's musical productions.

Time passed and I hadn't heard much about him, asking how he was in passing if I ran into his mother or his old staff. I remember hearing that he gave up soccer in seventh grade and decided he was going to wrestle. He ended up winning the "Most Outstanding Seventh Grade Wrestler" on his junior high team, although he had a losing record. His coach said that he was, "the only wrestler I ever met that cried while he kicked someone's ass." He had such a drive in everything he did and it was often visible that he was struggling with some greater force while trying to succeed, as if he was fighting against himself and his thoughts. Regardless of his internal battles, he always seemed to find a way to excel at whatever he decided to put his mind to.

I had read in the local paper that he even won a contest held by the famous Hershey Chocolate Factory in Hershey, Pennsylvania. He and some of his peers in his Special Interest program beat high schoolers in a competition involving creative and cost-effective ways to dispose of the burlap sacks the cocoa beans were shipped in. He actually created an entire Microsoft PowerPoint presentation before anyone was using this specific technology in his area. He and his peers even brought back a trophy that sits in his old middle school to this day. I was very proud of everything he was achieving. I felt like, in a small way, I had helped him become the young man he was becoming. It turns out, years later, that pride was not something he was able to experience, always believing that there was more to be done.

By eighth grade, he was the lead in the school play, the captain of the wrestling team, and a first chair clarinet player. He was a straight-A student and also ended up winning "Most Musical" for his class superlatives. He appeared to be a happy and confident young man with loads of potential. He had overcome everything that was thrown his way and made the best out of every bad situation he faced. However, as I found out soon after he started his freshman year in high school, his exterior in no way matched his interior. I was shocked to find a referral for him on my desk in early 1999.

After everything I had heard about his success in multiple endeavors, I never imagined that he would be

31

falling apart again, now almost 16 years of age. He had been demonstrating obsessive thoughts and mood instability during his first high school wrestling season. I knew how much he wanted to be called up to the high school team and sure enough, he beat out a senior for the 103 pound spot in the lineup. Prior to the start of the season, it was documented that he weighed almost 120 pounds. He had lean muscle and barely any body fat. He was able to make his weight for the first few matches but apparently he began weighing in at the mid 90's, close to ten pounds under what he needed to be. His coaches told him multiple times to take better care of himself and encouraged him to eat more than he was.

This is really the first time I noticed the level of obsessive thinking he was capable of. It turned out he was running three to four times a day and barely eating any food. He even told me that he would chew food up at school and then spit it in the trash can "just to taste it." Regardless of all the support he was receiving from the older wrestlers and coaches, he was unable to stop his decline. This was the first, but surely not the last, time that he was unable to finish a wrestling season.

No matter how much he improved his conditioning and technique, he was unable to improve his mentality. His worries rose to the forefront of his mind and soon he was spending more time with the guidance counselor than on the mat, or in the classroom.

His self esteem continued to be a concern when we finally met up that winter. You would never have believed everything he accomplished by looking at him. He appeared emaciated physically and exhausted emotionally. He had little to offer in conversation, but it was obvious to me how frustrated he was with the direction his life was headed. He wanted so badly to prove to everyone that he was tough. I believe that is why he stopped playing soccer and started to wrestle.

It is also at this time that he stopped participating in musicals and gave up playing the clarinet. He literally gave everything he had within him to be not just a wrestler, but a great wrestler. What he failed to understand was that he was never able to achieve greatness in this sport due to the strain he put on himself. He was unable to recognize his achievements and focused solely on his shortcomings and mistakes. This became another theme I noticed in him as we continued to work together throughout his life. It seemed that no one treated him nearly as bad as he treated himself.

January 4th, 1999 @ 0800

Student is a 15 year old Caucasian male. Alert and oriented x3. Currently denies Suicidal Ideation (SI) / Homicidal Ideation (HI). Student is not receiving any psychotropic medication treatment and still has no mental health diagnoses. Suggested seeing a psychiatrist to mother prior to Student leaving. Possible onset of mood and personality disorders developing. Obsessive thinking noted in referral per school guidance counselor. Eye contact remains poor, often burying head in hands. Tension observed in clenched fists and jaw. Observed as having a blunted affect, showing little emotion on face or in body language. Physically, Student was observed as possibly below healthy body weight. Will consider referring Student to internist for physical examination. Cheek bones prominent. Assessed Student's thoughts on physical appearance. Student verbalized no concerns with current physical health and stated "I need to maintain my weight for wrestling. I am in very good shape." Student denied any pressures from coaches or peers concerning weight loss, claiming, "Most of them are telling me

I need to eat more. This has nothing to do with them." Per the referral, Student has not attended practices since leaving the team during Thanksgiving break. Has been unable to attend practices during time off from school and has been reported as being unable to get out of car during attempts to attend said practices. Extremely tearful and combative per mother, although no physical violence or threats of self harm have been observed. Continues to offer little during questioning, a behavior noted in a previous meeting during which time Student was also under a great deal of stress. Attempted to assess Student's current state of self worth. Student did verbalize feeling like a "pussy" due to current inability to participate in scheduled wrestling practices and competitions. Student verbalized a continual frustration with the wrestler who "took his spot" and reiterated throughout our meeting that, "I am a better wrestler than he is." Discussed the importance of maintaining both physical and mental health in order to reach potential in current endeavor. Student showed signs of denial during this period of time, refusing to admit that there were any health concerns. Discussed current routine. Student stated that he runs approximately 3-4 miles prior to getting ready for school, eating either a granola bar or a health shake (shake consists of banana, peanut butter, skim milk, and ice cubes). Attends scheduled classes, as well as an extra gym class during free period to run more before eating lunch. Verbalized lunch consisting of minimal amounts of fruits or vegetables, and admits to chewing other foods and spitting them out into trash. Attends practice after school in which Student states running anywhere from 1-3 miles before a physically intensive two to three hour practice. Upon returning home, Student would eat meals separate from family, often lower in fat, and run once more before doing school work and going to bed. Based on Student's comments, this occurred five times a week, with competitions on Thursdays and Saturdays. Student did admit to exercising intensely on Sundays. Student may possibly be suffering from an eating disorder. Appears to have a preoccupation with weight and a possible paranoia, in regard to gaining weight/not maintaining current weight. Became defensive upon suggestion of changing routine and diet to improve current physical/emotional state. During this period of time, Student was observed as agitated, looking up from hand and raising voice in frustration with topic of discussion. Suggested continuing weekly or monthly meetings and consumer refused. Upon being picked up at the end of appointment, same suggestion was made to mother. Mother verbalized being open to the idea of scheduling more frequent appointments, however Student adamantly opposed.

Louis Bianco RN, CPS - end of visit note.

It was the first time I found myself genuinely worried about him and worried about his family. This once gregarious and bright child was now closed off, barely speaking unless spoken to, fragile physically, and obviously, at least to those who truly knew him, suffering mentally. I discussed the situation with some of my peers as I made my referrals to his primary care physician and our team of psychiatrists. During my brief follow-up, I found out that he did actually go see a physician, who ran blood tests and scrambled to find any signs of physical abnormalities that may have been causing this complete change in character. Because releases were signed, I was able to look at the lab results from blood work, and it seemed as if they found the streptococcus bacteria in his blood stream, claiming that he may be a carrier. The doctor explained in his note that some people are carriers of Strep and it may be the cause of the onset of his fatigue and depressive symptoms. I never heard from him or his family for almost two years following that meeting, and assumed that he was not going to take me up on the suggestion to see me more often. I could only hope that the recent findings in his blood work were remedied and he was once again going to right his ship and continue to grow into the man we all knew he was meant to be. Part of me hoped for this because I could see the hardships this was causing him and his family. Part of me hoped for this because, as I have stated before, I felt a slight responsibility for him.

I was proud of myself when I knew he was flourishing, and I surely doubted myself as he began to fail. I thought about all of our interactions since I met him when he was in first grade. I began to wonder if there were signs that I missed, if I somehow was leading this family down the wrong path. Mental health in general was not as prominent then as it is now, especially in children. We had to be very weary about diagnosing youth because it is difficult to differentiate a symptom from an age appropriate behavior. Kids are continuously growing and learning how to deal with themselves and their thoughts during their formative years. They may be hyper or whiny simply because they are kids and nothing more. I was always taught not to rob a child of their childhood by overstepping my boundaries in regard to assessing symptoms of illnesses that usually won't even carry any weight until 18 years of age or older.

And yet, as I sat and reflected upon our interactions, I found myself questioning the advice that I gave his parents as far as how tough to be on him and what to expect. I worried about the times I told him to "toughen up" and said things were "not that big of a deal."

During my Peer Specialist training, we were taught so much about the concept of the consumer being right about themselves. I feel like I may have immediately taken a role of knowing what was best for him simply because he was young. Had I done him or his family a disservice by not taking his concerns as seriously as he was? Am I somehow responsible for his current state of mind? I prayed each night that the lab results would lead them to the answers they were seeking.

Ultimately, those prayers were not answered. Hope is a funny thing. We talk so much about its importance in the mental health profession and try our best to instill it in those we work with. But in reality, it is merely a concept.

I am in no way trying to undermine the necessity of hope.

I have seen the power of hope first hand in those that I worked with over the years. People down on their luck, with nothing left to believe in but hope, have made such incredible strides towards recovery. Far be it from me to discourage anyone who says hope is a key ingredient in battling back from the hardships that life presents to us, but hope is not always enough. Simply hoping that something will get better is not enough to prevent it sometimes. This was the case with him. I'm sure he was hopeful. I'm sure his family was hopeful. I know that I was hopeful, and yet, things still got worse. Far worse than any of us could have imagined.

Chapter 4: The Storm

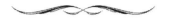

It was just a few days after New Year's Day in what was now the year 2001. I hadn't heard much about him in over a year. I remember looking in the paper to see how his sophomore campaign was going in wrestling. I never saw his name, but I also didn't hear from any of his staff or his family regarding subsequent breakdowns in his health. I continued to try and convince myself that we "fixed him" somehow. We found the problem, treated it, and now he was back to his normal self.

I didn't think much of the fact that I never saw his name in the paper, especially because it was now his junior season, and his name once again was popping up in the sports section. He never received his own article or anything like that, but when I read about the scores from his meets, I noticed that he was winning quite a bit. I remember being so proud of him yet again. He was such a resilient young man. No matter how hard different situations seemed in his life, he fought. He rebounded. There seemed to be a refusal to quit within him. I had heard that he broke his thumb prior to his most recent season starting, and yet there he was, overcoming the obstacles set before him and succeeding. I was shocked the day I got that phone call, just a month or so after his season started.

I don't remember exactly how I reacted when I picked up the phone that day. The news sounded so catastrophic I felt like I was in shock. It was his mother, she told me he was in the emergency room at one of our local hospitals. I couldn't see her face, but I heard in her voice that this was a very serious situation. I started to panic after she seemed unable to answer some of my initial questions and I rushed to the hospital to see how he was doing. When I asked her where I needed to go once I got there, she had already hung up the phone. I threw on my coat and rushed to see him. The entire drive was a blur.

I walked into the ER and remember telling myself to remain strong. This is not an easy profession. Sometimes I think that the consumers forget that we, as professionals, are humans too. We experience fear the same as anyone. Regardless of our knowledge of how the brain works and ways to control emotional responses, we are fallible creatures just like anyone else in the world. I took a few deep breaths after the nurse showed me where he was staying. Once I gathered my thoughts, I slowly walked into his room.

The first thing I noticed was how quiet it was. His mother and father were sitting in the corner of the room, consoling each other. I looked to my left and there he was. His face and body were covered in superficial cuts. There must have been one hundred or more. He was in a hospital gown that was covered in blood as it laid over all of the open wounds. I knew he wasn't in an accident because of the precision and symmetry of the cuts. He had done this to himself. I think I just stared at him at first. I had so many things I could have said to him, or even to his family, yet I was so taken back that I froze.

"Get out, I don't want you here," he growled.

I had never seen such anger in him. I thought back to my conjectures about his possible rage within. It was real, and when I looked in his eyes, I saw that he no longer had control of it. He then started covering his finger in the blood from one of his injuries and wrote "I hate you" on the bed. His mother was asking him why and his father appeared to be growing agitated with his careless and barbaric behaviors. I removed myself from the room and gestured to his mother to come speak with me in the hallway. I immediately apologized when she came around the corner. I gave her a hug and she began crying again. Her shirt sleeves were overflowing with used tissues. I'm sure that there were plenty of techniques I could have used in my skill set to attempt at calming her down or giving her some sort of peace. As I was thinking about the different tools I was taught for situations very similar to this, only one question found its way out of my mind and onto my lips. All at once, my curiosity superseded my responsibilities as a professional.

"What happened?"

There were so many ways I could've handled this better, I mean, I was the professional. I had dealt with crises before, a lot more than I'm sure his parents have. Why is the first statement I made a question that could possibly create negative emotions in someone who is already probably petrified after what they have experienced? Regardless of my beliefs that I could have handled the situation better than I had, I just needed to know exactly what I had asked. What happened?

Is this really the same kid that I worked with? The one who made hilarious movies for his school projects? The one who carelessly made others smile and laugh without hesitation?

That couldn't be him. He didn't look like him. He didn't act like him. I wasn't even here for five minutes and he was already mean to me. The kid I met wasn't mean to anyone, even when he was down. I needed to know more so I remained quiet following my question and allowed his mother to gather herself before she answered my query.

She told me she didn't know every detail. According to her, he stayed home from school after he begged her for some time to rest because he wasn't feeling well. She began telling me she should've known better than to leave him by himself and I immediately expressed that none of this was her fault. There was no way of knowing he would have done this to himself, regardless of how he was feeling or any changes in his behavior.

She continued with the story and stated that she had gotten a call from her oldest daughter around lunch time. According to her, he had called his sister following his self mutilation. She could hear him begging his sister not to call an ambulance, but to no avail. It was now in the hands of the adults and this young, confused teenager no longer had any power as far as what was to be done next. Although he argued and pleaded that everything was fine, I remember feeling thankful that he didn't escalate the situation to something that required police involvement.

I guess, in that moment, as I was beating myself up trying to figure out where I went wrong, I was looking for some sort of positive amidst the chaos. She continued with the timeline as she knew it and explained how he was loaded into the back of an ambulance right in front of their house, on the same road where he learned how to play basketball. His sister must have followed behind in her car and waited with him until his mother showed up. She had to leave work, so did his father. I can't even imagine what they had to say to their respective employers. He was already checked in by the time they arrived. His mother then asked me one of the hardest questions to answer in my field of work.

"What do we do now?"

I started to freeze again. What do they do now? I wasn't sure that I even knew how to answer that question. I decided to be completely honest with her and tell her exactly that. I explained how he had set something in motion now, something he was unable to undo. I tried to give her forewarning on the lengthy process that was about to occur due to the choices he made. I could only assume that he was going to need psychiatric care, be it hospitalization, medication, or both. He still didn't have an exact diagnosis, but that was almost sure to change based on where he was. He was in a hospital. He had very little choice on what was going to happen next. He was either going to agree to the care that was suggested to him or be involuntarily committed to an institution where he

47

would have even less say in the course of action moving forward.

We both knew at this moment that there was something much more severe than dormant strep in his bloodstream. He was exemplifying symptoms associated with mental illness and it is as if the dam had broken. The flood gates were officially opened.

I requested some time alone with him so I could do a brief assessment for his documentation. I wasn't sure how he was going to react to seeing me one on one, but I still felt I owed him my time, away from his family, in case there was anything he wanted to disclose without their knowledge. I now had to be very careful however, and I made sure to tell him that prior to us talking. I explained how people in my profession are not allowed to keep everything confidential, specifically if he had thoughts of harming himself or others. It was my responsibility to all the parties involved, including him and myself, to report any of this if he ever admitted to it. I was somewhat surprised that he agreed to meet with me. I told his parents to go grab something to eat. Who knows when they had eaten last, or if they were even hungry?

I had so many questions for him, but I remember in my training how important it was to let him lead the conversation. My desire to have my questions answered was not as important as his possible necessity to express himself. I had to fight the urge to simply ask why. His demeanor changed slightly from agitated to frightened and tears welled up in his eyes. He never actually cried though, I know I would have if I was in his situation.

He explained to me that he had done everything in his power to express that he wasn't doing well. He was visibly frustrated with the fact that no one believed him. His mother would check his temperature to see if he had a fever and when he didn't, she and his father would insist he went to school. It started to get so bad that they threatened to call a truancy officer on him if he didn't get out of bed. He stated that he had no other option to prove to others that he was in pain. Here we are again, trying to prove something. He had quit performing in musicals to prove he wasn't gay. He had quit soccer and replaced it with wrestling to prove he was tough. It was never enough for him to believe his own truth.

He needed to show others how real his truths were, and he often did this at the cost of himself. It was never more real to me than it was that day. I truly don't think even someone as intelligent as him knew how serious his actions were that day. Even if he did, there is no way that he could have been prepared for everything that followed after one bad choice was made by an exhausted and confused teenager. I asked him once more if he was thinking about hurting himself anymore and he shut down. I was able to recognize that we weren't going to get too far on that night, and he had spoken enough to me that I was able to do my note, but so many things were left unsaid. I still wanted to ask him why. I had such a difficult time trying to grasp the idea that someone like him felt so alone and desperate. Don't get me wrong, I understand that even something like this could've been worse, but I couldn't help but feel pity for him and his family. I couldn't help but feel guilt either. Had I failed him? Would I ever get to work with him again? I know it wasn't the right time to doubt myself, but like I said earlier, we are all human. I had a tough time sleeping that night.

January 9th, 2001 @ 1930

Patient is a 16 year old Caucasian male. Currently has no mental health diagnoses and is not on any psychotropic medications. In emergency room on suicide watch following self injurious behavior (SIB). Observed as having over 100 cuts on head, neck, arms, and torso. Cuts symmetric and superficial, no stitches needed upon arrival. Affect blunted. Patient currently denies SI/HI but verbalized "I hate my life." Offered little during one to one interaction while parents were in room. Spoke with patient while parents ate dinner. Patient still offered little insight into situation. Shared some details regarding crisis. Patient verbalized using a broken shaving implement to cut self. "I took the guards off my razor. I just wanted to bleed. I didn't plan on so many cuts. I just couldn't stop." Questioned Patient about current status of school, wrestling, etc. Patient refused to engage in any further conversation and stopped responding. Unable to attain specific physical data from facility (i.e. weight, lab results, EKG, etc.) but Patient appeared malnourished and emaciated. Upon speaking briefly with parents prior to departure it was determined that neither parent was home while crisis occurred. Patient verbalized feeling sick and requested time off of school. Waited until alone before self-mutilation. Patient then called sister who found him on kitchen

51

floor covered in blood. Sister immediately called 911. According to the sister, Patient became verbally aggressive and did not want to be taken to hospital in ambulance. Was noted as belligerent while talking on phone with different family members prior to ambulance arriving. Per family, Patient did consent to ambulance transportation and no police intervention was necessary.

Louis Bianco, RN CPS - end of visit note.

Chapter 5: Not Otherwise Specified

I followed up the next morning with his mother. He had been taken to another hospital and been placed under psychiatric care for the first time in his young life. This was the first time he received a mental health diagnosis. He was only 17 years old. Usually, in the mental health field back then, you had to be 18 years old before you got full fledged diagnoses, but based on his current symptoms and behaviors, the doctors diagnosed him as follows:

Mood Disorder NOS (Not Otherwise Specified)

Anxiety Disorder NOS

53

Borderline Personality Disorder Traits

Obsessive Compulsive Disorder Traits

Basically, he was now on the fast track to having multiple disorders as an adult. Mood Disorder NOS can become a few different things in adulthood, although, at this time in his life, it appeared that all signs were pointing at Major Depressive Disorder, or MDD. Anxiety Disorder NOS just becomes GAD (Generalized Anxiety Disorder) or something more severe associated with anxiety. Saying that someone has traits of the other disorders listed above basically means that they are demonstrating the warning signs of said disorders, but require further assessment or are too young to receive official designations.

Concerning the OCD traits, the doctor explained to his parents that he suffered more from obsessive thinking than he did from any compulsions that followed due to the thoughts. He wasn't a checker or a counter, symptoms that his parents were more familiar with regarding OCD. The doctor also believed he had something known as Seasonal Affective Disorder. This was believed to be caused by the increased darkness in winter following daylight savings time. It was the belief of his doctor at this time that his depressed mood and subsequent behaviors were caused by a chemical imbalance that occurred due to lack of sunlight as winter set in.

The following 48 hours were life changing for him and his family. No one knew what to do or how to act. He was started on "psych meds" for the first time in his life - antidepressants and anti-anxiety medications to be exact. The doctor also required him to wake up hours before breakfast and sit in front of a lamp that emitted artificial sunlight. Between the morning routine and the sedating nature of his new medications, he found it very difficult to follow the regimented and strict schedule on this locked psychiatric unit. He was soon falling asleep in groups or not getting out of bed on time.

His punishment? Not being able to have any visitors. I remember that this specific unit had not yet even created an adolescent unit. His roommate was in his mid 40s. There was an 80 year old woman with dementia who often dragged her suitcase up and down the halls yelling to herself during social hours. He was not comfortable being there. Some of his family members weren't comfortable visiting, but his parents always did. He didn't always want to see them, but they always showed up.

Just from my professional experience, I feel the need to describe what a standard, basic, run of the mill psychiatric facility consisted of. First of all, everyone is locked in. Although one is free to travel in and out of their room, all patients are locked on the actual unit 24/7 with some facilities allowing for outside time with permission from a doctor always being necessary. Some people act up to the point that they must be physically restrained by the staff in the safest possible manner. If the physical restraint is not enough to restore order, chemical restraints become available, often in the form of an intramuscular shot. Patients meet with their psychiatrist daily, and on weekends, they meet with whatever doctor is scheduled to work. The doctor assesses the effects of current medications, as well as discuss behaviors documented by staff from the previous day. Other things documented by staff are amount of sleep, food intake, vital signs, and bathroom habits.

There is also something called 15 minute checks. This simply means that every 15 minutes a staff walks around and documents the whereabouts of each individual patient on the unit. During periods of sleep, the staff is to assess that the person is breathing prior to continuing checks. At night, they walk around with flashlights. Other than that, every facility structures their days differently, usually revolving around group therapy and one on one meetings with the various staff.

Group therapy is when a therapist or mental health professional holds a session that is approximately an hour long with all of the patients on the unit. Some facilities divide the groups up based on cognitive or behavioral limitations, others do not. Some facilities make groups a requirement, others make them optional. Often, as was in his case, there is a behavioral based point system in place with rewards such as visits and fresh air offered as a reward. Go to a group, get some initials on your score sheet, qualify to see your parents during your inpatient stay.

As a professional I can say, even when optional, attendance is documented and often, missing a group is used against you in one way or another. In one's moment of complete detachment from necessary life sustaining behaviors, it remains a responsibility to achieve self control.

In his case specifically, I was unable to visit with him in the morning. They continued to wake him up at four in the morning to sit him in front of a lamp. They said the absence of adequate sunlight was causing this fall from grace. He was heavily sedated due to the newly prescribed medications working their way into his body and mind. He was chemically unstable they said. He needed medications to avoid cataclysmic failure, we told him. He slept through breakfast and got reprimanded. He always tried so hard to do everything right. Follow every rule. Believe every authority figure. He was so scared because even he didn't fully understand his current reality.

We believe confident conjectures are facts when we are most frightened. Those who speak from an authoritative and informed position must choose their words carefully because the uninformed and fearful are listening to everything you are saying. What he and his family were being told wasn't all fact, but it was spoken as such and, in this moment, he and his family needed to believe the experts. No one else knew what was happening. This was a legitimate problem. All parties agreed something was broken. But was it unfixable?

It wasn't long before he wanted to leave the "psych ward." Between being a teenager on an adult unit and being punished for a sedation that was created by the very regiment he was required to follow, his mental health was not improving. Throughout his life he was humbled. A talented, attractive, gregarious young man must not get too big of a head. This was the way he was raised. This is the way those that raised him were raised. Those around him were not aware of how important their favor was to him. They truly had no idea how attentively he listened to every word and struggled tirelessly to be what those around him said they needed. He was not conceited.

In fact, his self-esteem was dwindling at a frantic pace. So while those around him, including me I'm sure, made sure to keep his head out of the clouds, we buried it deeper into his living hell. We clipped the wings of a bird that never even believed he could fly. Now he sits alone, covered in dried blood, surrounded by strangers. Surrounded by more adults explaining to him why what he was doing wasn't enough for the "real world." Haha, the "real world;" don't make me laugh. As if reminding him that he was defective was going to increase his ability to improve his position! All we were doing was over-warning the already over-cautious, threatening the scared, isolating the lonely.

I listened a lot during this period of time. I endured criticism and misplaced anger from his direction. He attacked my weaknesses and all I was doing was trying to help. I knew he needed me. I always told myself that the hatred he was spewing was not his, nor was it directed at me. I did believe that the rage existed, however, and the only way to be free from it was going to be to rid himself of it through emoting.

He said that no one loved him. Nothing was ever enough. He was unable to see what people were trying to give him because he was not getting what he needed. He missed out on outreached hands looking where there were none. He shut down. If he didn't want to talk, he was insanely disciplined. If he wanted attention, he was masterfully manipulative.

He was wielding a power that no child should be responsible for and was given no instruction manual. It was far beyond the mind of an adolescent to control. Many adults never experience it, and even fewer handle it as he did. He appeared to continually swallow hand grenades and endure the pain internally. The shame. The guilt. In his mind and heart, he knew it wasn't all his fault but he took it all himself. He was unwilling to give this to anyone else, yet unable to control it himself. Damage occurred during periods of weakness.

Relationships were tested. His life, and the life of everyone around him was different. He tested boundaries, but he always backed down. He wanted so desperately to be heard, but he was afraid of retaliation, so often his attacks were discrete and strategic, and only heard by those willing to listen. He was very quiet in his attacks, but very precise. His greatest target, the target in which he dealt the most emotional and physical abuse, was himself.

Looking back to that period of time, I'm mad at myself for not realizing how strong he was. Although it was not a healthy thought process, he was killing himself to protect those around him. He was putting up walls while crying for help. He was scrambling for anything that might work because he was actively failing. The fear in his eyes told his truth. As human beings, we innately protect. We also innately warn. Discord in relationships occurs when we ignore warnings, often to protect ourselves from boundaries within which we are not comfortable.

Imagine a dog barking at a person. If the person is smart, they give the dog more space. On the other hand, if the person is insecure, they may want to prove to the dog that it shouldn't be barking. In this instance, the person continues closer to the threat to feel better about themselves, not to help ease the dog's agitation, misguided or not.

It is important to recognize a warning regardless of whether or not you think it's rational. Recognizing warnings is one of the greatest protective measures one can take. But, as mentioned previously, inaccurate perceptions of a warning can actually elicit the behaviors all parties are trying to avoid. These types of situations appear to be prevalent in the mental health world, often occurring when an uninformed party assumes a leadership role that they are unable to handle appropriately.

At times, this self appointed "leader" becomes more scared than the person who was suffering initially. This was the case for my young friend. Everyone was scared. He was the child. The adults, having no experience or understanding of his specific situation, assumed responsibility with an internal hesitance but an external urgency. In attempts to fix what was broken, they relentlessly attempted to find answers while he refused to talk. Because he didn't have the answers, they could not figure out the solution. Because they said he was sick, he was removed from the team working to heal him.

None of us listened to him as much as we listened to the "experts." We created a dynamic that actually bred illness. We told him to pay more attention to warning signs and red flags, as defined by us. We told him that every one of his unique character traits somehow explained why he was damned for the rest of his life. And, being the loyal, idealistic, shame ridden teenager that he was, he allowed others to treat him as faulty.

As a third party, I can honestly say that every time I received a call from him I assumed I was going to hear about another disaster. I always assumed I was going to be entering into a crisis. Soon, everything was a crisis. But was that because of his fear, or because of the fear I, and the other "experts" projected onto him? Can we blame a teenager for believing what his doctors and parents told him was happening?

He ended up in a different hospital. This hospital was further from his home and further from his family. This hospital, however, had a child and adolescent unit. Doctors trained to work with youth, specifically. There were times allotted specifically to stay caught up in school work. His peers were much closer to his age, if not younger. At least now, his surroundings made more sense to him. He still didn't want to talk when I went to see him. I was told by one of the staff that his grandfather traveled over two hours to see him daily, and then drove two hours home. I also heard that during the actual visit, he ignored his grandfather.

He refused to talk to him.

He refused to look at him.

He demanded that he leave.

It turned out that his grandmother, on the same side (maternal), suffered from bipolar disorder during her adult life. His grandfather may well have been the person who understood him the most at that moment. His grandfather may possibly have been the person he treated the most unfairly. No, that was his mother - the daughter of said grandparents, the oldest of four, the woman who watched her mother deteriorate, the child who assumed adult responsibilities too early because of the mental illness her mother had.

His mother had seen this before. She did everything in her power to avoid this becoming a reality for any of her children. And yet, there he sat; unimpressed by the visits from neighbors and clergy, uninspired by notes and letters from friends and family. Although the word love was continuously thrown around verbally, he was not feeling it. Realistically speaking, loving and well-intentioned are two very different concepts. In this instance, he was surrounded with well-intentioned individuals who had no idea how to love him, nor did he understand how to love himself.

A loving environment requires an understanding of the members within it. Ultimately knowing those around you allows you to give them the safety and security necessary to grow. A well-intentioned environment still consists of good, caring individuals. However, because the needs of each person is specific to them, just intending to do good by others isn't enough, especially if your good is actually their bad.

There are circumstances in which one's needs defy what you understand to be reasonable. If your love is unconditional, you adapt and adjust. Learning is loving. Advising, warning, cautioning, reprimanding, teaching, and the like are well-intentioned. Without learning, there is no love.

In the dynamic involving a child and an adult, like the one I found myself in with him, the adult feels that they know best. In truth, they most likely do. The part they must learn is how to deliver their message so that it can be received in a non-threatening manner to the child. What is threatening, you ask? That is precisely my point. It must be learned. Answers within relationships exist within that relationship. The truth is there, somewhere.

My age had nothing to do with his needs. He was telling me what he needed. I was telling him he didn't need that. I didn't think he needed that. I decided for him because I am the adult and he is showing that he obviously cannot make any important decisions about his life at this time. I was well-intentioned. The staff were well-intentioned. His family tried everything they could to love him, but only some actually did. Inversely, he only loved some. Fear ultimately dictated who chose to love and who could only remain well-intentioned. Neither is a bad choice considering the countless relationships that exist without even common decency. Regardless, he wanted certain people to do more than they were doing. He wanted to make the well-intentioned love him. There were times when he believed he needed this. Feeling so strongly, in fact, that he actually used words such as neglect in describing his past. He held us all to the standards he held himself. The standards we told him were expected. The standards we told him defined normalcy and emotional health. After all, that's what we told him he needed to do in order to get better. But did any of us even do what we were teaching him was healthy?

Maybe his expectation existed because we taught him to practice behaviors we didn't practice. Maybe we were only well-intentioned. For example, we taught him assertive communication, but assertive communication only works with those who can receive it as assertive. The majority of the people around him heard assertive as aggressive. His honesty was threatening because it wasn't pleasant. His verbal assessments of his reality allowed those who didn't agree with him to tell him he was wrong! Not because they knew any better than he did, but because he was wrong by default. He was mentally ill. We have since learned much more about the differences between mental illness and intellectual capacity.

He continued to use the techniques we told him were necessary, and it created more distress. This, and many other examples like it, were now defining his life.

You can't control your thoughts, but don't even think certain ones. If you do, if you even think it, call this expert and get help immediately, you are in grave danger. And remember, you can't control your thoughts, so don't beat yourself up.

The mind of a gifted child was now flooded with tapes of conjecture being spoken as fact. A bright young man somehow was trying to figure out how to march to everyone else's drums. The most amazing piece of this story was the way he still found ways to be successful for short periods of time. It was as if all of the random noise in his head sometimes struck a harmony that made sense. He stayed caught up on all his school work during this entire ordeal. He lost his best chance at a deep run in the state wrestling tournament. He was having the best season of his high school career and, unfortunately, he could not get that back.

Wrestling was so important to him. His entire life he was labeled as the baby. He cried because he felt everything intensely. All jabs felt like hooks. He was proving something to himself as much as he was proving it to those around him. This was a very driven and intense human being. This was a very intelligent human being. What we learned from wrestling was that this was also a tough human being. His work ethic within the practice room was rigorous and admirable. He often drove himself to tears just to push to a gear few are brave enough to enter. He didn't start until 7th grade and ultimately became a four year varsity starter.

His coaches didn't understand him, but they tried. They allowed him to continue to try and fail. They never shut their doors. He did not have the medals or even the record to be held in high esteem, but if you were on his team, you knew who he was. Possibly because of how he worked, possibly because you watched him self-destruct. There will always be talks that the excessive exercise and weight loss created a perfect storm during puberty leaving him with some sort of neurological-deficiency. It was always important to him, however, to stress that it was all his doing. The coaches never demanded from him what he demanded of himself. He also claims to have survived his life long suffering because of what wrestling taught him about himself. He doesn't blame the sport; he is thankful for it.

The proverbial buzzer had sounded, but the fight had just started and he knew he could push himself to do what was necessary to survive and ultimately win. He channeled his energy and continued to grind on his academics.

Chapter 6: Misdirection

He had enough support from his high school teaching staff during the summer and began summer school at his home at the end of the school year. It was very important that he graduated with his twin brother and he refused to fall too far behind. His teachers were wonderful. He was not always in the best of moods and there were a few times he cancelled scheduled appointments, but those people continued to put themselves out for him. I have such a high level of respect for the effort they put forth to help this young man find his way to a high school diploma. He worked hard for them because they worked hard for him. They worked hard for him because he worked hard for them. Think about it.

This is a concept that meant a lot to him. It was how he decided who was safe to him and who was a threat. He learned at a young age how much he could improve himself with effort. He believed it was a choice to improve. He always made that choice for those he loved, and felt loved when he saw that type of effort from others. He saw it from his coaches, and now he saw it from his teachers.

He graduated with his class in 2002 with academic honors. He won "Best Sense of Humor" in his senior superlatives. In a graduating class of over 650 students, with the complete fall from grace he was experiencing behind closed doors, he remained the class clown. The picture in the yearbook shows him with a sling on his arm for a shoulder injury he exaggerated in order to avoid failing once more at the sport he loved. Comedy was his smokescreen, but as any half good con man knows, misdirection was a necessary skill for survival.

He really did know how to make people laugh and, unfortunately, he was willing to do almost anything to get the response he was looking for. He especially liked to degrade himself and, unfortunately sometimes, others.

He always allowed others to do the same to him. He let people spit on him or punch him in the head for money. As I look back, I too found myself laughing at his pain as he creatively camouflaged it with humor. We all missed the subtle cries for help he was making, as he appeased our most basic needs with physical humor and a quick wit.

When he finally asked for help in a way that we took seriously, it was already too late. Somehow, when he started pretending again, we all fell under his spell once more. We must have just wanted to believe deep down that "this time" was the time that he was actually better. I sometimes wonder if he was just being our jester because of his understanding with our realistic inability to solve his problem.

In spite of all the trials and tribulations, he graduated with high grades. It was another smokescreen. We, as adults, saw high numbers on a piece of paper and encouraged him not to undersell his ability. Not to settle. No to underachieve.

This meant applying for and being accepted to a "state school" to continue his education on the college level. It was important to his parents that he get a college education, and his father worked especially hard to help provide that. This was how his father expressed his love, through hard work and fiscal discipline. His father denied himself of many things in order to maintain financial stability for the family, and my young friend was hell bent on not letting his father down.

It was his initial intention to attend college and study to become an elementary level school teacher. I remember conversing with him prior to his departure and hearing what sounded like sincere excitement in his voice. It seemed, at least at that time, possibly again because of his ability to pull the wool over our eyes, that he was finally over the hump. Once again, we, the observers, could not have been more wrong. Not only was he continuing to struggle with his own thought processes, he was now immersed in a world that was, for all intents and purposes, set up to perpetrate and even worsen a condition that was already spiraling out of control.

For a young man with such a low self-esteem heading into this experience, the idea of finally being able to experiment with drugs and alcohol actually intrigued him. Up until this point, it had only been a traditional vacation week for newly graduated teenagers -- one last hurrah before strapping on the thinking caps again for college, a trip to the beach for a week with only his friends, surrounded by groups of other teenagers from around the country with the same intention: party! With minimal experience and understanding of the effects that such substances had on him, especially with the plethora of medications he was putting in his system daily, he experimented with liquor. Although his behaviors did change, it was not enough for his immature mind to comprehend as a warning sign. He continued to drink heavily well into his freshman year of college and began experimenting with marijuana as well; yet another sign we missed until it was too late.

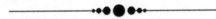

Chapter 7: Drowning

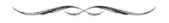

I had always appreciated that he listed me as an emergency contact, and yet, I dreaded this as well. I found myself having minor bouts of anxiety every time I heard my phone ring at hours I considered late. Unfortunately, as is the case with many of us who fear the worst, it happened. I received a call from his dormitory's RA midway through his freshman year. They described to me his condition as they had discovered him. According to authorities, non-legal, he was discovered in his dorm room conscious, but extremely inebriated with an empty medication bottle at his side. The pills, 20 plus, were in one hand, and a half empty bottle of coconut rum was in the other. His roommate had recalled that he was on the phone earlier with one of his sisters, distraught, angry, and ultimately lost. Although we had seen him in states where he was willing to harm himself superficially, this was the first real time that his behaviors were escalating towards lethal. Obviously underage, it was ultimately decided that he would not be punished by the school or the law if he agreed to attend therapy with a psychiatric professional. I volunteered to provide the counseling part; however, he was also required to see the university psychiatrist. I drove down that weekend to meet with him.

February 15, 2004 @ 1000

Patient is a 19 year old Caucasian male currently diagnosed with a Mood Disorder NOS, BPD (borderline personality disorder) traits, OCD (obsessive compulsive disorder) traits, and generalized anxiety. Currently receiving medication therapy for mood (SSRI) and irrational thought processes (antipsychotic). Verbalized little therapeutic effect from current medication regimen but also states that medication is being taken according to prescribing doctor. Denies SI/HI however meeting is taking place due to incident involving threat to overdose on medication while inebriated. Observed as

78

disheveled and unkempt, with eyebrows barely visible. States no recollection of removing eyebrows, however, per write up from staff, Patient removed own eyebrows during drunken stupor. Responses to questions brief and affect is flat with only visible emotion at this time being agitation and/or frustration with current situation. Unwilling to discuss idea of alcohol use increasing due to stress stating "I feel this way every day of my life, people just don't want to believe me." Patient had verbalized reaching out to coaching staff of university wrestling team about suicidal ideations. He continued to describe how the head coach scoffed at him and made it clear that he, the coach, was not someone to get support from. Patient verbalized disdain for the idea of receiving treatment while attending the university but realized the alternative, possible underage drinking charges and expulsion, as worse. Patient did not consent to sister being reached for her recollection of said incident. Made numerous suggestions on possible behavioral changes that may improve current state of cognition, all of which were refuted by Patient, who ultimately continued to question how much longer our meeting had to continue. Explained time requirements to consumer (one hour minimum). Patient became verbally aggressive during second attempt to discuss the idea of alcohol being a catalyst of recent behavioral decline. Received consent from Patient to share results of interaction with college psychiatrist; however, Patient refused to sign any consent to share information of situation with family. Also important to note decision to move Patient to a more supervised floor in dormitory.

Louis Bianco. RN, CPS - end of visit note.

It had appeared that he had done enough to get back on track, at least superficially. Based on our previously described interaction, I was sure that he was going to continue to drink. He verbalized to me much later in his life that the only way he felt capable of decreasing his alcohol consumption was through his usage of marijuana. Marijuana, during the time that his life was falling apart, had not yet been seen for its possible medical benefits. Let it be known, even from the eyes of a professional, he appeared to handle his burdens much better while using that specific substance. Regardless, and we will talk about this in much greater detail at another time perhaps, he knew it was illegal and he ultimately was unable to find comfort using something that provided him relief from his affliction because of that fact.

A recurring theme in his ongoing struggles - the things that helped were not seen as appropriate by those around him, and the cycle of refraining from effective interventions only drove him further into darkness.

Going into his sophomore year of college, he continued to attain the highest of marks in his education -- 4.00 across the board. He was also humiliating himself publicly to make people laugh. Additionally, he was sexually promiscuous and he was also wearing sunglasses because he gave himself two black eyes with his own fist. He was feeding an ego with an endless appetite for immediate gratification, and then experiencing high levels of self loathing. It was one of his addictive cycles.

At times, looking back, it seems we put too much emphasis on certain criteria and completely ignore others. It was as if we convinced ourselves that his grades were an indicator of his well being. He remained in excellent physical shape, running sometimes twice a day and working out in the gym as well, while smoking cigarettes daily. He was able to move off campus for his sophomore year and shared an apartment with his friends, most of them from his high school, and some he met during his freshman year at the university. General education classes were over and the curriculum now found him working directly with children in the university's elementary school classroom settings. Although he excelled in such situations, he was growing increasingly anxious with his new workload and soon began skipping classes and avoiding such scenarios. He was never worried that he would lose his temper around children, in fact, most of his life he was excellent at communicating with youth. However, he was continuing to drink at night, even during the week, and found much more solace in the party lifestyle, forsaking his responsibilities for what he believed was peace of mind. He would never work with children while intoxicated so he just chose to forsake his dream for his addiction.

This, however, came with a price. He stopped attending his education classes all together and instead continued to pursue the subjects that kept his interest. In this case, it was sociology and film. Knowing that his absenteeism was going to catch up with him quickly, he continued to attend and maintain high marks in said classes but ultimately crashed and burned when he ran out of excuses for missing the other parts of his curriculum. As this unrealistic fantasy he created came to a screeching halt, he once again found himself agitated, overwhelmed, lost, and out of options. His father received a call halfway through the first semester of his sophomore year from the university psychiatrist. He had cut his entire body up again, superficially, and was sitting in the doctor's office wearing a blood soaked white tee shirt, eyes bruised and expressionless. Although he denied it at the time, he has since been able to admit that he knew no other way to deal with the extreme levels of agitation teamed with the complete inability to function on an "age appropriate" level. He was never going to unleash his rage on others. To him, there was only one person strong enough to endure his true rage; himself.

At that moment, given all of the work he put in to rise out of the ashes he was in after he crashed and burned the first time, he found himself in almost an identical situation, albeit with very different circumstances. How can this happen? How can someone with his level of intelligence, and now years of therapy and medication, end up in the very situation that we had all tried our best to avoid? I will save my more advanced explanation for the end of this specific story, but let's just say, it was not ALL his fault, although the choices he made were his own. Let me explain this further:

He had now spent multiple years of his formative life being told to watch out for symptoms and possible warning signs that a crisis was on the horizon. He spent years being told that he was broken even during periods of success and he was being told these things by medical professionals and valued adults in his life (doctors, parents, teachers, etc.).

I believe that such messages being sent, even with the best of intentions, can have a negative effect on any human. Telling someone they are broken and cannot be truly fixed for the rest of their life is a narrative that is difficult to remove from one's mind, especially a mind as active as his.

Amidst all of the accusations and labels, the expectation that he remained a kind person who made reasonable decisions remained a requirement. This led to increased guilt and shame when he made poor choices, something many young people, mentally ill or not, do. Years of this type of cognition soon caused him to, at times, act outside of his own moral code as some sort of protest towards life. The expectation that he immediately figured out what he was going to do next remained a pressure he was experiencing internally and from others. The paradox of the world he lived within was maddening.

Think back to that concept of "Social Disability." He is what we were telling him:

"There is a defect in how your mind works, but think clearly."

"This isn't something you can get rid of, you're sick."

"Why can't you figure out what you are doing with your life?"

"You better be really careful this doesn't happen again, and this will happen again."

How was it that all of these statements were being said to the same person? How was he expected to make sense to anyone who believed he had a defect before interaction? Why did we expect him to keep fighting when we kept telling him he lost?

These are just a few questions he used to ask me. Hearing it from a teenager, I often disregarded or deflected a lot of this as some type of "outburst." I would immediately assume he was just upset and trying to figure out who to blame for his current misfortune. I never realized he was trying to explain to me the hell he existed in. Surrounded by good people who "try to help" with good intentions. To him, trying to help had nothing to do with trying to fix. Helping was believing that the pain he was describing was not made up or due to any one decision he made when he was not even old enough to describe the death sentence they presented his life as. To him, helping was believing that he knew what he was talking about after realizing he spends his life thinking about everything.

What happens when you introduce unnecessary fear into a gifted brain?

What happens when you tell someone born to soar that he can't fly?

What happens when you try to keep him humble when he already hates himself?

He just needed us to listen to him. What he was presenting and verbalizing as his state of mind had remained unchanged and consistent for years at this point. He used to tell me to imagine drowning surrounded by people just yelling from safety "swim harder" or "you know how to swim, I have seen you do it before!" People watched him suffer and just offered him advice from a safe distance. He made it seem like he had spent the majority of his life treading water ... just "holding on." It all sounded exhausting.

The level of darkness he experienced in his life, past and present, was only matched by the glow of the light he saw ahead of him. His mind was the cause of his suffering and the reason he kept fighting. I am blown away at the thought of how many times he may have already tried to tell me that he was sinking.

Why didn't I see it when it was happening?

Was it because I thought he was too young?

Was it because of my own preconceptions?

It must have been, no matter how many ways I try to justify my decisions. Hindsight is 20/20 as they say. Regardless of what we should have done, his father drove him out of college. Out of the frying pan, into the fire. We were foolish to think this was over. It was just starting.

Wednesday, May 4th, 2004

Patient is a 20 year old Caucasian male. Denies SI/HI, however Patient does state "I hate my life." Suicidal protocol may be necessary although Patient contracts for safety. Poor eye contact. Clothing and hair disheveled. Flat affect. Currently on antidepressant medication, anti-anxiety medication, antipsychotic medication. Visible superficial cuts bilaterally on face, limbs, and torso-SIB. Both eyes are ecchymotic. Refusal to engage in conversation about incidents leading to crisis, giving short answers or non verbal gestures. Attempted to find out more about previous statements regarding suicidality. Patient grew increasingly agitated stating that he has "no intent to kill himself." Suggested that Patient see current psychiatrist as soon as possible as well as therapist. Patient requested to leave session early. Discussed briefly and session was completed in 20 minutes (60 minute session).

Louis Bianco RN, CPS - end of visit note.

Chapter 8: I Will Survive

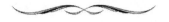

I never valued his words or realized how much he thought before he spoke. I was always trying to pinpoint which symptom he was exhibiting and whether or not he was in control of his emotions. If he cried it must have been because he had depression. If he didn't like his life, it must have been proof he was suicidal. I never thought back then about what he was saying. His behaviors had proven that he was going to fight this illness no matter how juvenile some of his antics became. He just hated life at that time, and I would have hated it too. The alarm that goes off when he would say things like this to mental health professionals was always triggered. We taught him early on to be honest about his feelings and when he started speaking we told him he shouldn't say such things. His words were honest. Our words were driven by what we have learned in school, and our own belief in the assumption that we know exactly what someone means, even if they don't say it.

My ego interfered with our communication. He was reaching out for help and we, as professionals, were attaching symptoms to his requests. This is not to say he wasn't at times spiteful with his words. Trust me, in the times in which he was creating chaos, his words were venomous. They had to be. He was making "mistake" after "mistake" and wasn't even 21 yet. He almost didn't graduate high school and now he was dropping out of college. I kept thinking to myself when I would hear about him, "now what?" It wasn't until I got older and spent more time in this field that I realized all of his bruises and proverbial broken bones came from trying and failing. No matter how much preparation and attention he paid to his own safety, his crashes were violent and often unexpected. He hated his life and yet he kept dusting himself off and trying over and over again. His words were true and indicative of an overall negative state of mind, but his behaviors were saying I will not give up.

The conversations continued to improve because of all the material he was learning while being hospitalized. This gifted brain began perfecting its communication skills with the promise from us that that's what he needed to do to be "normal." He improves, starts communicating as we taught him too, and we then quickly pick apart everything wrong with his verbalized thoughts, never needing to share our own thoughts orally for the same criticism. He spoke his truth and we explained to him the parts he was wrong about.

I learned a lot about myself working with someone like him. The more I realized how hard he was trying, the harder I tried. Mental illness is ugly. Our inability to completely understand it is dangerous. Our "one size fits all" mentality of treatment is a death sentence, but so is radical acceptance. He didn't want to be enabled, he just desired to be heard. Our inability to listen is unacceptable. His story is one in which the diagnoses perpetuated the illness. The help we were giving him was not necessarily the help that he needed.

He spent the next few years of his life working odd jobs. He seemed to find some peace in manual labor choosing employment at landscaping companies and local nurseries. He helped his brother in law with construction and HVAC work. He worked at day care centers and summer camps. He even coached the junior high wrestling team of his alma mater. He continued to write music and started recording songs at his home and sharing his CDs with his friends. The first song I heard from him was with the background music of the legendary disco classic "I Will Survive":

"Survive" (early 2000's)

At first I was afraid,
I was way scared.
Could not find my way,
And I didn't care.

I gave up all hope,
Sliding down this slope.
I couldn't even get good news out of my horoscopes.

I fell down and I couldn't get up.
Fell off and I couldn't get back on,

Now I'm gonna put my mack on.
Combat with the past, cut the slack,
No more "whack son",
I'm gaining on the pack son.
I'm sorry too Miss Jack-son.

This road to recovery,
And discovery,
Search inside my soul to see,
If I can find a better me.
There better be
Ways for me to kill my inner enemies.

They better see
That this is the last guy they are gonna beat.
They hungering,
Gunning for new ways to get inside of me.

Oh hide me please,
From my disease.

Who holds the keys?
To the history,
Of my misery.

It's a mystery,
Why I wish to be stable,
Willing and able.

Turning the tables,
Happiness to me is just a fable.

A fairy tale.
Good prevails.

First I need some wind to come around,
And blow my sails,
A gale.
Cast me off into the right direction.
Steer me clear away from my dissensions.

Deny perceptions,
Apply corrections,
Attain perfection.

Give love and get some.
Give more and then some.
Someday the answers will come.
So will more questions.

I need interventions.
New inventions.
No more of my true cruel intentions.
Did I mention apprehension?

The only way to triumph is through my own
comprehension!
No dissension.
I bet ya, I will survive!

I'm gonna stay alive!
There ain't no illness in the world that's gonna take my
life!

I got my arms out wide,
And I'm ready to fly.
I got my two fists raised and I'm ready to fight!

Come on God, now I'm ready,
Give me your best shot!

It's been four long years and I still ain't dropped!
You need more than just depression if
You think you're gonna stop this.

All you've done is slow me down.
Knock me on the ground.
Make my head spin round and round.

A few scars and a few black eyes?
Not yet.
A pair of eyes that forgot how to cry?
No sweat.

Run me through your gauntlet.
Treat me like your puppet.
The harder you make it the stronger I get.
You can't stop me.

And one day I'll wake up and pay off my debt.
One day I'll stand up and none will forget.
When I opened my eyes,
With a smile on my face,
And I no longer felt that my life's a disgrace.
I'll be back to my family,
Back to my home.

Showing them all what I did on my own.
When their words couldn't help,
And their hugs couldn't heal.
That's the cards I was dealt,
When my heart couldn't feel.

The day is coming up.
The day is drawing nye.
And ya'll better believe me,
Cuz this ain't a lie.

I might look like a quitter,
Like I lost my drive.
But know in your hearts,
And soon you'll realize.
This game might be over,
But I never lost… in overtime … I will survive.

Chapter 9: Functioning Appropriately

Starting to slow himself, he settled down for a little and with that settling he healed some of his wounds. The problem with him was that he often found comfort in discomfort. This is a phenomenon that is now prevalent in our society, even in individuals without a mental health diagnosis, yet also a behavior that led to him receiving a diagnosis. Think about it… I find this type of paradox in a lot of people who have suffered trauma.

Yes, I mean trauma. We often associate trauma with whatever we perceive as worthy of the designation. War and post war effects, for example, are just our society agreeing on what they think trauma is and then closing their minds to its existence outside of those circumstances. But not all soldiers have guns, and not all wars are fought on foreign soil. Fearing for one's life every waking second changes a person. Never feeling safe, and safety is a need, changes a person. Unwanted situations alarm our nervous system into panic insistently. The only way to survive this, is to continually absorb it and remain on task. No one is born to withstand such torture, let alone continue on, fighting for your life during all waking hours. Long periods of this mentality are the reason we survive but not without its negative effects.

Humans are products of conditioning. Behaviors, statements, feelings, over a long period of time become part of our mental makeup. Unfortunately, not all of these conditions work in society. Stimuli continue to trigger the survival response, trust deteriorates. The line between friend and foe blurs and soon, conflict is created, possibly even unconsciously, because it makes more sense than order.

Panic is a comfortable discomfort because it is at least familiar to the victim. Situations that involve a survival mentality are sought out because they make more sense and within the perception of "making sense" is safety. I would never dare to speak for anyone who has experienced something I haven't. I myself have a great deal of respect for the bravery of soldiers. I also believe in the severity of Post Traumatic Stress Disorder (PTSD) and the effects it has not only on the afflicted, but the loved ones around them. I am just saying, that if we studied the behaviors associated with the illness, we would see that trauma expands far beyond just one single event. Trauma breeds trauma. We are wasting our time deciding whether or not someone should be feeling something based solely on our opinion. However, the behaviors of someone who has suffered trauma are more visible if we just assess more than we decipher.

I am as guilty as anyone of this. I didn't see that he was traumatized. He had what I considered a good life and loving family. There is no way he could have experienced or been experiencing trauma, based on my perception. Unfortunately, my perception was inaccurate.

He continued to drink excessively. He never touched alcohol in high school. He abused it in college. In his early adult life, he became a functioning alcoholic. Nothing during the week, then fifths of liquor all weekend, even stretching to Thursdays. He was the life of the party at the beginning and the carnage at the end. Caution was never exercised in the presence of anything that helped him escape himself. Alcohol, marijuana, nicotine, and caffeine being used to create the facade of stability. It was always obvious to me how good or bad he was actually doing by how much he was consuming. The excess in which he consumed liquor specifically, was a sign that he was giving up on trying.

We thought he was doing fine. He was working and going to school. He had a romantic partner and plenty of friends. So what if he gets drunk all weekend. Who doesn't? What a delusion we have created as a society; this idea that excessive alcohol consumption is acceptable because everyone does it - this societal removal of responsibility if inebriated, even though getting drunk is as much of a choice as any made under alcohol's influence.

His drinking was a symptom of his system failing. His reality was one so miserable that he hid from it with a central nervous system depressant. That's right folks, alcohol is a CNS depressant, literally shutting everything down to feel a buzz. The more you drink, the slower your body and brain become. Drinking in excess just to feel better meant that he still hadn't shut his body down enough to find peace when he was slightly drunk. He usually lost to the drink, passing out and often urinating in his sleep, as an adult. Is that supposed to be the funny story he talked about next week at work? Or maybe he would have to apologize again to those that he loved for his behavior and cancerous words.

It was officially a problem, but he had a job. He was working. He had a girlfriend. He was doing good, we told ourselves. All of the boxes that proved someone was functioning in life were checked. Sadly, however, his battle with alcohol wasn't over yet, though he began trying to get it under control. All that actually meant was that he became even better at being a functional alcoholic; an alcoholic hiding under the guise of socialization and happiness, both the opposite of what a depressed person would do. Yet, one more reason he felt like a walking contradiction.

Chapter 10: Calling

The path his life took began creating an undeniable urge to become a mental health professional. I originally wrote "undeniable desire" instead of urge, but the fact is, that wouldn't be true. He was already exhausted from his life and the pressures of being "more" than he was comfortable with. Yet, so much of his life was spent learning about cognitive change and the power of self, that he refused to settle and seek comfort in accepting a self he wasn't ultimately proud of. It was all so fascinating to me. His evolution, for lack of a better term, within the mental health system amazed me. Even though he continued to suffer, the way he chose to behave during that suffering never passed a certain line of morality, allowing him to "save face" in a society he desperately wanted to become a part of.

At this point, he could not attempt achieving another four year degree due to his finances and recent cataclysmic failure. He was very fortunate to have a quality local community college that offered a nursing program. He had remembered seeing nurses on the psychiatric units he received care from. He remembered that I was a psychiatric nurse. Less than ten years had passed with two life altering crises at such a young age and he was once again pushing himself forward. Amidst broken relationships, weight gain, alcoholism, and increasing social impulsivity, he was trying yet again. The nursing program he got accepted into was the most competitive program in the area at the time. The workload was heavy and the information was dense. Even within the pre-requisites, he found himself needing to maintain discipline and focus that many thought he had lost.

He began his life again, driving himself to and from class everyday, and driving to different hospitals for "clinicals" (required education days working on actual

105

hospital floors with an actual patient load). This kid who didn't even get his driver's license until he was 19, was now a full fledged commuting college student with a part time job in his mid 20s. The person who once had complete meltdowns under intense pressure, was now facing his greatest fears to achieve his goal. We again got a glimpse of the person we believed he was. We so easily get lulled by the idea that everything is going to be okay because he always gets back up. The idea that someone is "better" creates a false sense of security in onlookers. He was always fighting.

He was using every ounce of effort he could to hold himself together and maintain a passing grade in a very demanding pursuit. He was under constant scrutiny and was, for the first time, feeling like he didn't belong in this class. Others were smarter and more confident, skillfully breezing through all of the requirements and procedures. He was doing excellent paperwork and showcasing a high level of bedside manner, but he wasn't acing tests. He sought extra help. He toiled and sacrificed hobbies to stay afloat. But again, he was near failure. In his second semester, he sat down with the director of the program and quit. This was now a recurring behavior at this point in his life.

I waited for the phone call. He said he was going to go back to full time with the landscaping company he worked for, but I knew he was hurting inside and that a crisis was looming. Then I caught up with his mother and she told me he broke his foot. What we didn't know at the time, was that he actually tried to do this, slamming a dumbbell on his foot repetitively in hopes that it would keep him from working.

He was failing, again, but this time he was hiding more. He didn't want to go back to another hospital. He needed to keep pushing. As the hiding increased, the behaviors intensified. The drinking and monetary spending increased. He started staying up all night and sleeping all day, but we saw a smile. It is amazing how that smile was enough to fool us. He knew what we were looking for as far as symptoms, so he made sure not to show us. He put on another mask to make us feel better. I wonder how alone he felt, assuming full responsibility to fix something he didn't break, to have full accountability for words and emotional control. He had to learn everyone else's language because no one was willing to learn his. The more I thought about it, the more I feared impending doom. I never got that phone call though.

I have to admit, when I heard the news that he got himself back into that nursing program, I couldn't believe it. He only took one semester off. Within that time, meetings with professors and the director of the program were scheduled. Out of classroom work was completed as well as the necessary administrative tasks necessary for reinstatement. Just like the last time he faced a crisis, he fought, and again, so did the educational staff. He rose up, and this time, he had recovered sooner. His pattern had changed. His endurance and stress tolerance had increased as well as his recovery time. Soon, he was back into the program with a fire that we have only seen rarely within him. He began working as a secretary at a psychiatric facility in the city while he continued his education.

In the winter of 2008, almost ten years since his life changed forever, over five years since he recovered and graduated high school, over four years since he dropped out of college for the first time, and over a year since he dropped out the second time, he graduated nursing school. I went to his graduation to support him only to see that he didn't even attend the ceremony. Then I found out he failed his licensing exam the first time. I knew how hard those tests were and I certainly didn't have the anxiety that he did. Yet again, in his truest fashion, he sulked, recovered, pushed, and achieved. On the second attempt of the NCLEX exam, he passed. Officially an RN, he signed on with the psychiatric facility he was already working for, now as a psychiatric nurse. He went from patient to professional, before the role of Peer Specialist even existed. Oh, and he was living with a therapist he worked with at the hospital. He had moved out of his parents house when they weren't home to avoid confrontations.

It was one of the few times I believe he was actually proud of himself, at least concerning his licensure. I thought to myself, how ill is this person? Look at what he has done. He knows more about himself than we know about the science. Here is this driven, passionate, young man succeeding in the face of all of our labels and warnings, abiding by all the rules we taught, showing up to appointments consistently, taking medications as prescribed, still fighting his own demons because our treatments were not meant for him, and graduating nursing school.

Even as I write this, I find myself inspired by his toughness. Broken and put back together more times than anyone deserves and still so young, refusing to be held back from his destiny. Were we standing in his way under the guise of necessity? Perhaps we were more delusional than he was. It was such an ugly process to watch, but that never stopped him. He was hell bent on figuring himself and his life out and unwilling to lose. He understood that the system was imperfect, but still believed it was necessary. That is why he chose to start working within it.

He was just running a different race than those around him. Endurance was incredibly important in this pursuit, as he had to watch all of his peers sprint by him. This tested his self esteem. He felt lesser than. There were no awards for his greatest accomplishments. What he did was expected of him to prove health, anything less than our construct of normal meant illness. At a time when he was actually excelling, we felt like he had finally just caught up. We couldn't have been more wrong. He had done everything we had done, yes. He was now living with his fiancé, making good money from his full time job with benefits.

That's "normal."

That's "healthy."

But for who?

Who creates these universal definitions of such important words as normal and healthy?

This life that he had finally achieved was not his truth. It was the mask that kept the most people around him comfortable. When those around him were comfortable, he wasn't scrutinized, meaning he too was comfortable. It was what we told him he needed to do to be "better" in OUR eyes. How often do we negatively label something just because it is foreign to us? The comfort of putting something unknown or confusing into an understood

111

context is a luxury of those that label, not those being labeled.

In mental health, it is our responsibility as professionals to do right by our consumers. They arrive lost, we must try our best not to lead them astray. They are seeking our guidance and direction and are listening to what we suggest. If we don't know what we are talking about, we cannot continue to matter of factly hypothesize. He was dealing with being the patient in a broken system and working as a professional to try and improve it at the same time!

In a short amount of time, he went from medication nurse to charge nurse. He became the lead on the team that intervenes with agitated consumers and any dangerous situations involving conflict as well (Crisis Team Leader). He worked with adults, the elderly, and even the youth. He was excelling professionally, but failing socially. This is not to say that he didn't make lasting relationships with his peers, but he continued to be careless with his behaviors and his heart.

At that time, the stigma of mental illness was far worse than it is now. No one knew that he had a mental illness because he hid it. He was in charge of a psychiatric unit, he wasn't going to lose all of that talking about his past. He had to listen to staff talk poorly about consumer behaviors and, at times, demean the suffering of those they didn't believe. He never opened his mouth. He was hurt and also scared of losing everything he had worked for. It was more of a culture than any single individual.

I know I worked with well-intentioned caring mental health professionals my whole life. The majority of my coworkers did their best to give consumers the best chance to try again in life. But I would be lying if I said that everything I saw was recovery-oriented. The power structure that he experienced as a patient still existed when he arrived as a professional. I believe that we are so afraid of disorder as professionals that we sacrifice compassion for control. Trust me, I understand the necessity of control on a unit. I have been in the trenches my whole life. It is dangerous at times. I can understand, to a degree, the idea of never feeling safe, but that was only while I was on the clock. He had to do it on the clock, and off. He was juggling multiple personas and exhausting himself in the process. He kept up his act as long as he could.

Chapter 11: Overqualified

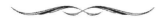

The marriage only lasted for a few months before he divorced his wife and moved in with an assortment of family and friends. He and his wife had bought a house together early in their marriage and he did not fight to keep it. He knew he needed to get out of the relationship and he tried to do it with as little conflict as possible. At the height of his professional career he was bouncing around from house to house sleeping on couches and living out of duffle bags. He continued to consume alcohol, finding numerous relationships, both casual and romantic, in settings where he was inebriated. The necessity for immediate gratification remained, the ego now seemingly insatiable. He still got drunk, he just stopped blacking out. He also continued to smoke marijuana whenever it was available.

If it weren't for substances, he wouldn't have had any friends. A lack of relationships is a sign of isolating. Which is a sign of depression. Possibly a behavior exhibited by someone with borderline personality disorder, right?

This is an example of the thought processes we created within him. This is how we programmed him. It was important that he showed us what we needed to see. The part we missed was that he needed to dumb himself down to be what we wanted from him, and he chose alcohol. Even that, with all the medications he was taking, was not enough to bring him peace. The majority of his adult life, he felt guilty and disappointed. We believed the lie he was living, for our own comfort. There was always so much more happening in him than he ever led us to believe. He had us all fooled, or maybe we were just willfully ignorant.

Financial and social stabilities were priority, and he was finally achieving it, moving his way up the proverbial food chain due to his work ethic and understanding of human behavior and interaction. Although he didn't admit his past, he used the empathy he learned to connect with patients no one even wanted to say hello to. His confidence in his ability to perform was always different then his self esteem. He knew he was capable of completing tasks well. The difficulty lied more in the toll even seemingly menial tasks took on him and the confusion of those around him when he tried to explain his tribulation. Relationships were constantly being strained by misunderstandings or the inability to empathize. He even met another woman who worked with children and lived with her for almost two years. However, as we often see in those who pretend, sustainability was not possible.

Soon, his sick time began to dwindle at work. Arguments at home intensified. He began searching for something to help him escape, but he feared being drug tested so he abstained from marijuana. During that time, synthetic marijuana was being sold legally and did not show up on drug tests. The simple idea that he was allowed to do something that he felt was so helpful was

117

actually a high point during his descent. What he didn't know, and what many around him were unaware of as well, was the incredible danger those substances invited. What once had appeared to be the perfect compromise for him, soon became one more bane of his existence.

He abused this substance, sometimes sharing it with friends. On more than one occasion, he found himself spending hours on end with friends, who panicked because they believed they were dying during their high. He smoked it multiple times a day after work shifts and spent hours recording freestyle raps on his laptop. Other than his close circle of friends, he kept this toxicity a secret from loved ones.

If anything, his spiral accelerated and soon he found himself in the human resource office with no more medical leave and an inability to work. He had to either quit or he would have gotten fired at that point. An easy decision to observers it appeared, "just go to work and you can keep your job". A consistent discussion he had with all of those he spoke with about his dilemma. How do you describe the phrase "I can't" when all signs point to more than enough ability? The medications were not

118

working, and now, neither was he. Whether we understood it or not, his "I can't" actually meant he couldn't.

He quickly found another position, with even higher pay and increased responsibilities. He even had his own office and nameplate. During orientation, his boss told him she didn't think he was going to be a good fit. The next week he got confronted and reprimanded for documentation that was "too long and thorough." His peers poked and prodded to break him. They did not want him there. He was already much weaker than he let anyone know. During his daily hour long commute to work, he was crying on the phone with his father, wiping his tears away in the parking lot before walking into his office.

At one point, he deescalated a young teenage girl who was actively harming herself with a sharp implement. He actually got disciplined for this, and was written up for overstepping his job description. He was punished for a believed usage of marijuana until his drug screen came back clean. How many false allegations can one person endure? Rumors of misinterpreted quotes and

119

fabrications soon swelled his head as he found himself under attack with no defense.

He broke, at work, in front of peers, superiors, and subordinates. The tears could no longer be held in, the rage was too great to contain in this toxic environment. The perfect storm had officially touched down. His weakness was exposed. He cared deeply about people's perception of him. He was destroyed by others saying things about him that were not true. That was the opposite of the character he believed he was portraying and beyond that. Values and morals were being called into question. He hurt himself in his office with a staple and quickly told a coworker he trusted. They walked him out to his car, so as to not alarm the children. He knew that he would not allow the kids to be aware of his poor judgement, but remained almost in awe that he had such a lapse of judgment in a professional setting. He took medical leave, not being fired by his company.

Unable to show his face to those around him, he quit. Now out of a job, he began scrambling. He picked up random part time nursing jobs. He worked at a clothing store and even tried night shifts in a factory that made lawn equipment. He asked local business owners if they needed janitorial help or a dishwasher, but his resume often excluded him from work he knew he could do. He was constantly told he was overqualified for the work he desperately needed now to survive.

We used to believe that he just needed work that wasn't as mentally taxing, but the "easy" periods of employment were even shorter than when he was on the front lines in a psychiatric facility. His girlfriend had since lost her patience with his erratic behavior and repeated failed attempts at recovering from the most recent gut shot life threw. She said she couldn't do it anymore. She ultimately left him. He was feverishly trying to right a ship that had already sunk.

He was unwilling to admit defeat and wasted countless breaths trying to convince those around him not to give up yet. There is no way an observer can understand that someone is running for their life just by watching them. He was trying to survive and maintain employment and stay present in a relationship. He was incapable of such responsibilities; he was drowning ... again. As he moved back in with his parents, he realized he was willing to do anything to rid himself of this madness; anything, even a new treatment he had never tried yet. It must just be the wrong medications, we thought to ourselves. "Let's do this (ECT) first and then change all of your medications again if we have to," said the doctor.

Chapter 12: ECT

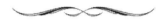

Sounds like a plan to someone willing to do anything. By the way, ECT stands for Electroconvulsive Therapy (shock therapy, you know, like in One Flew Over the Cuckoo's Nest). So what would compel a human being to willingly be put under anesthesia and allow a doctor to send electricity directly through their body by way of their brain? The concept basically is that this procedure aids in the resetting of all of the chemicals and neurotransmitters in the brain. The same chemicals and neurotransmitters that we believe become imbalanced, creating what we believe is mental illness.

Imagine the use of an AED on a person in the midst of cardiac distress or complete heart failure. The rhythm of the heart doesn't work right, so we shock the body to hopefully reset said rhythm. In mental health, there are still no diagnostic tests to pinpoint deficiencies in the aforementioned components. There is no real way to tell if the procedure works other than observation of behavioral or cognitive changes. He had studied up on the treatment as best as he could, and learned that there was a lot of success in those that were "medication resistive," a new phrase he began hearing from his treatment team.

He decided to set up an appointment with me to discuss all of his options following his departure from his longest job ever to date. He was once again unemployed. I remember being shocked at the sight of him, having not seen him in person for years. He was close to 250 pounds. His skin was greasy and he reeked of cigarette smoke. His hygiene was fading and dry skin was flaking off of his face. He looked more broken than I had ever seen him although I did notice his increase in ability to control emotion and verbalize what he was experiencing. He didn't yell as much. He didn't sit in silence anymore. He was suffering out loud, making logical point after logical point about how this could have been handled better in his youth. In the midst of another crisis, during a depressing and disheartening outpouring of sadness, I was able to recognize the improvements he was making.

I found myself wondering how many times he was going to have to create a different game plan only to fall flat on his face in the end. I empathized with him now more than ever before because I at least knew what it was like to be a psychiatric nurse. That in and of itself was enough to overwhelm even the strongest of individuals. He was doing all of that with medications failing, drug and alcohol addiction, a disintegrating relationship, and a realization that he still was not free from the darkness that was chasing him. Every piece needed to work perfectly and the very second one cog shifted, the entire machine malfunctioned.

This brilliantly designed, intricate system was still missing something. Another foundation built only to crumble under greater weight than one can ever fathom in preparation. As he grew stronger, so did his illness. The harder it became to maintain, the more reckless his behaviors became to disguise it. We found ourselves at a crossroads and an important decision needed to be made. I remember his increasing agitation with the imperfect science that was psychiatry. The role of lab rat began to plague his thoughts, and this was someone who was very agreeable throughout his life in regard to treatments.

He was always willing to try whatever was suggested because his ultimate goal was recovery. But how many times did we tell him what a medication was going to do only to have it fail? How many times did we justify our mistake with the infancy of our understanding?

This was a person who was just trying to be more than a professional patient. This was a life that we were basically playing scientist on, and because we had failed him to this point, we were now suggesting an even more invasive procedure. We were convincing him, and ourselves, that this was his mess to clean up. And once again, he ultimately trusted us.

June 10, 2012, 1200

Consumer is a 28 year old Caucasian male. Currently on antipsychotic and anti-anxiety medication. Presents as disheveled and unkempt. Consumer has gained a lot of weight.

126

Labored breathing and diaphoresis observed. Tearful. Appears to be under a great deal of stress. Denies SI/HI currently, however did verbalize altercation with significant other which involved the threat of overdosing with medications and alcohol. Consumer states he was just being manipulative and feels very guilty for his inability to control this impulse currently. Discussed suicidality further and agreed that more intensive treatment may be necessary. Observed small, superficial cuts on arms. Consumer verbalized a disappointment in recent SIB. "It had been a long time since I hurt myself." Verbalized helplessness. Continues to express a hope for future. Discussed ECT. "I'll try anything at this point. How in the world did this happen again? What have I done on this earth that makes me deserving of this? I have fought and scratched and clawed since I was a kid and this is still the end result?" Frustration noticeable in consumer's confession, as well as desperation. Made referral to psychiatric facility and consumer contracted for safety. "I'm not going to hurt myself, I just need help." Discussed alcohol and drug abuse. Consumer verbalized the cessation of synthetic marijuana due to fear of side effects and possible illegality. Continues to drink liquor but verbalizes an understanding of the risks. Consumer verbalized an attempt to decrease or cease his alcohol consumption. Continues to smoke cigarettes and is adamantly unwilling to stop smoking at this time. "It reminds me to inhale."

Discussed safety and treatment plans with consumer and girlfriend prior to departure. Also gave out paperwork on how to receive county assistance. Consumer is no longer receiving insurance from previous employer and has medications and possible ECT to pay for.

Louis Bianco RN, CPS - end of visit note.

I met him in the waiting room before his second of twelve treatments. His parents would always be there. He wasn't allowed to drive due to the anesthesia. He talked a bit with me about the treatment experience. The first thing he ensured me of was the care he was receiving from the nurses. He was actually receiving this treatment at the hospital where he was a charge nurse once; by doctors he attended report with. He was receiving care from nurses he stood arm in arm with during crises. Dedicated, compassionate, and efficient nurses, former co-workers, seeing him in a hospital gown, and working on him while he was unconscious. They were looking at him while electrodes were pasted onto his head and chest.

They were listening to his body convulse as the doctor sends electricity through his body. They were keeping him safe and alive in his weakest state.

Watching him panic as the reversal agent made him experience a conscious withdrawal while the anesthesia took hold must have been horrifying. He told me that nothing scared him more than knowing he was going to lose consciousness. It was in that moment that I realized how much he valued his mind. The same thing that has him here for this traumatic experience is the part of him he values the most; yet another paradox that unfolded during our time together. His life was full of them. I can't imagine allowing former co-workers to see me in such a compromised and vulnerable state. He truly was willing to do anything to figure this out.

If there is one thing you can say for sure about this kid, he put his money where his mouth was. To the uneducated eye, he appeared weak and fragile but anyone wise could see how much this young man was enduring. He never skipped an appointment. He was never late. He was scared as hell and willing to stare at that fear, face to face, just for a chance at peace. After twelve treatments, he was discharged, feeling weakened, but hopeful. This was it; life was going to be better from here. Little did anyone know at the time, the shock he received did not just wake him up, it woke a monster.

———————•♦● ●♦•———————

Chapter 12: Mania

He was almost 30 years old now, already over a decade and a half of suffering and fighting. Already over half of his life was dedicated to figuring these issues out as fast as possible.

As an adult, he had lived a life very true to the diagnosis assigned to him - extreme success, extreme failure. The highs were fulfilling yet fleeting and the lows left him scarred and disfigured. He was running from what he was trying to protect. His gift was his curse and his persistence made things harder. Yet, the storm had passed and he was still treading water. He was a survivor of yet another crisis. Now coming out of the wreckage with little damage other than a complete loss of short

131

term memory, he felt rejuvenated. He was ready to take on life once more, this time at a slower pace than before.

The pace of course, during any time of recovery, is incredibly important. Move too fast, and you find yourself in a situation in which you are unable to act accordingly. Externally firing on all cylinders, you can achieve the greatest of tasks, but ultimately, the speed is unmaintainable. Overwhelmed and exhausted, unable to stop in time, it is an accident waiting to happen. Move too slow, and complacency grows exponentially.

Procrastination leads to postponement, ultimately resulting in absence. Usually, this absence does not just pertain to the physical realm. Mentally, the absence of aspiration, integrity, dignity, and even capability will often lead to inability. Without being shown a finish line, it was now up to him to decide what pace would be appropriate. He continued to go to therapy and psychiatrist appointments. He got their input on what his next move should be. He spoke with his parents and friends. Ultimately, employment was the first checkpoint. He knew he wasn't ready or able to function as a nurse currently. He was still recovering from ECT. The benefits

132

show themselves slowly. Some of the side effects were brief, some lasting. He decided to pursue a different path this time and he set his pace.

Off he went, this time, with the belief that he was meant to be an artist. During his ECT recovery, he found himself writing lyrics and free styling more feverishly than ever. He was giving his projects more time and intricately weaving his messages about living with a mental illness into his songs. He never wanted to mention a lot of his suffering directly. His music was often more of a creative attempt to tell others what he was experiencing without making them uncomfortable. He still knew how to wear the masks. He was changing, however. He started working at the mall in a paint your own pottery studio. His hair was longer and he picked it out and walked around with a receding hairline afro. He was paying a studio producer now to help him make his basement recordings sound more professional. This was a new mask we hadn't seen from him in a very long time - the artist.

He had always excelled artistically in school. Whether it was drawing, playing musical instruments, singing, writing, or musicals; he participated enthusiastically and was quite good. This was the part of himself he thought he needed to hide during the more insecure moments of his youth. It was something he ultimately could not ignore. No matter how much money he made in the field of healthcare, no matter how successful he looked to us on paper, he was suffering. In order to avoid that suffering, he submitted somewhat to the idea of a truer self. We watched him dance and smile again. We danced and smiled with him. He was not depressed. We knew that. He was actually becoming manic. We didn't know that. As is a theme of this narration, we saw what we wanted to see.

He looked better to us based on what we perceived better to be. Even when talking with him years later, he admits he didn't realize it was happening either. His ego was ready to feed once again. He became more deliberate during his attempts to get his fix, but his behaviors were never more risky. Social media and heavy alcohol consumption in social settings, helped him meet friends of friends with the intention of physical intimacy. He never forced this issue, but he was persuasive and cerebral, as well as patient.

He believed that his ability not to act on impulse made those around him more impulsive. Sexual promiscuity with people from old jobs, ex-girlfriends, and even others in failing relationships became his narrative, forsaking his integrity yet again to feed. He ignored his conscience to feed carnal needs. He justified his behaviors based on the lies he repeated as if to convince himself his exploits were acceptable. Never seeming more confident, he was actually more desperate than he had ever been. The upward spiral is as dangerous as its downward counterpart, it's just easier to watch in its early stages.

This is not to say that he was sleeping with everyone he met. Hyper-sexuality is a symptom of mania, the high side of bipolar. Although he was more promiscuous in this state, he still experienced feelings of remorse and guilt. He still believed that emotions were important and was never able to sink into the mindset of "it's just sex." One night stands were not on his agenda, and instead, he just began dating people that were obviously not right for him. He invested in his partners emotionally and allowed himself to be vulnerable, all the while meeting his more basic physical needs in the process.

He never cheated on any of them, although he did find himself in situations where some of them may have been cheating on others. He took more risks as far as public displays of affection, and took to social media to pronounce his love for people he was involved with for less than a year. Loved ones and friends alike would question some of his choices, only to be met with his anger, often acting as if he was personally attacked by such questions. Even still, it appeared easier to label him as a serial monogamist than someone experiencing mania.

Soon, he was making music videos, performing his original songs live, and living everyday as his alter ego, his monster:

Monster

Verse 1
First I start to sweat,
Both armpits wet.
A heart tachycardic,
On your mark, get set, GO!

136

I transform;
The man form,
Of cancer.
Until I look like a Rancor,
But handsome.
I'm a monster!

Every time I'm given a rhythm,
Like a magician, a prism
On all considered musicians.

And then POOF!
Tada, ya'll oblivious spitters.

The dark wizard,
Cold heart killer,
Magnificent villain.

Veins bustin' out my suit now.
Longer tooth now.
Incredible Hulk,
With heavy bulk,
Makin' boo sounds.

Beware of my mind,
My thoughts are perverse.
You jocks will be cursed and dropped,
In a coffin or urn.

Chorus
It goes Errr, Errr

137

Doctor Funkenstein created me!

Howwwllll,
Full moon, werewolf baby teeth.

Mwahahah,
I need an artery to bite,
Artery to bite.
Jojo's hungry gotta feed tonight.
(Repeat)

Verse 2
Gotham city is ruined.
I am The Joker plus Bane.

Toss in The Riddler,
Cuz my lyrics will just,
Drive you insane.

I'm blindfolded and
I'm flyin' the plane.
Pilot beside is dyin,
Because my rhymin's,
Freakin fryin' his brain.

Ghostly,
Host with the most beats.
Freestyle fanatic,
Look closely.
Pyromania toasty.

With words I be rippin' like Jack,

138

Like Vlad, stickin' my staff,
Inside of your stupid ignorant AHHHHHHH!

Don't give me a flask,
Or any flack, I'm violent.

This is simple,
You're witnessing some Jeckel and Hyde SHHHHH!
A hybrid.
Of bipolar designs collidin',
With the likes of,
Jason, Freddy, and Myers.
O'Doyle Rules.

I'm that bully in school,
King Kong with my beast dong,
Screwing these fools.

You are simply misconstruing the truth.
Cuz there is nothing that should scare you more than,
Monster in the booth!

Chorus
It goes Errr, Errr
Doctor Funkenstein created me!

Howwwllll,
Full moon, werewolf baby teeth.

Mwahahah,
I need an artery to bite,
Artery to bite.

Jojo's hungry gotta feed tonight.

Bridge *(sung like Phantom of the Opera)*
Run and hide!
Here he comes!

Bloodshot eyes,
Near the cusp!
Dark Side Sith Lord,
Chessier grin.

Maleficent.
More desperate.
Not hesitant,
To let this gift take over me.

Verse 3
Please restrain me.
I will never go mainstream.
Unless my brain bleeds,
And then I write like I'm age three.

I won't refrain speech,
I won't be concrete.
It's abstract.
Mad Hatter flowin' beyond beats.

Get your wands please,
I'm he who shall not be named.

I brought a snake,

Evada Cadabra Snape!

Rotting bodies now decompensate.
As the zombies wait,
In a hypnotic, catatonic state.

God of hate,
Top primate.
Twisted prodigy.
Never wearing Prada G,
Demonic anomaly.

Probably, that's why I see a shrink.
And take pills,
Yellow, purple, blue, green, or pink!

Chorus
It goes Errr, Errr
Doctor Funkenstein created me!

Howwwllll,
Full moon, werewolf baby teeth.

Mwahahah,
I need an artery to bite,
Artery to bite.
Jojo's hungry gotta feed tonight.

Regardless of how careless he was with his life, he treated his creativity as precious. He constantly critiqued his own work, even taking projects down from the public eye (social media) if he felt it wasn't exactly the quality he wanted it to be. There were days when he felt everything he thought of or created needed to be shared, and days when he would delete everything he posted. His creativity was soon noticed locally and the music video that he had made with his friends was now on a progressive website dedicated to his home city. He was soon writing for this website and attending meetings with city officials and others grinding towards social improvement. His credentials didn't hurt, as he was able to expand the relevance of his cause with proof of education. This attention then landed him his first professional opportunity as an artist. He was commissioned by one of the city's local theaters to write a song for the end of their production about the History of Harrisburg. Upon his first visit with the cast and crew, he was offered a role in the show, along with guaranteed money. He took to the stage yet again, once the lead in middle school musicals, now a paid actor in his state's capital.

But his writing was soon inadequate per the website's owner and operator. It was too "stream of consciousness." He didn't space appropriately; technical criticisms. The theatre company, after milking him for all he had, questioned the choices he made on stage at times; more technical criticisms. It was as if his mask created the facade that he was trained appropriately. He was trained to be a nurse. His entire adult life was spent on a psychiatric unit, be it as a patient or a professional. He inserted himself into his community artistically in less than a year and quickly established local relevance. It blew him away, and also stifled him. He could not believe those that took him under their wing had such high expectations of him. He felt as if he begged to be taught but was never even given the chance. He used to say, "Teach me first. If I fail after that, get rid of me." He was succeeding on natural talent and instinct. Imagine the impact he could have had with proper training.

He continued to believe he could create his future on this path. He saw the pieces moving into place and planned his attack, but did not pay enough attention to detail. A failed video project for the website ultimately led to being completely ignored and denied further opportunity. Discomfort in acting classes and the feeling as if he was undervalued sent him away from theatre. Even a busted audio system during two consecutive live shows led him to question if he was meant for this life. The writing was on the wall. Money was tight and "real" employment was soon necessary. If that wasn't enough, he was unable to return to his previous job due to indiscretions. He was drinking less but smoking more cigarettes and marijuana, coffee and more cigarettes, medications daily, often two or three times a day. Flying by the seat of his pants, barely hanging on while traveling through life at a breakneck speed, we couldn't have been happier. He seemed content, truly, even if you had asked him. Again, mania is not necessarily noticeable in its watered down state, which is hypomania.

Hypomania is like a drug. It is a high disguised as a 24/7 personality shift. As someone who spent so many years feeling depressed, he loved this new mindset. He wasn't frivolously spending money he didn't have, he was still saving. He wasn't sleeping around, he was in relationships. He slept at night. His words remained impactful and still had meaning. He was writing feverishly. All of these were signs that he wasn't manic.

Often, we look for extremes to decipher how sick someone is, but those extremes are usually negative. Once someone is no longer able to function appropriately, we label them as mentally ill.

In his case, he was succeeding at maintaining employment and even volunteering. He was coaching wrestling with an old teammate and making digital art and video for the program's websites as well. He was speaking at local schools, trying to promote mental health awareness, long before it was the cool thing to do, before mental illness became trendy. He had realized the importance of mental health long before society even decided to care about mental illness.

He was sending emails to schools and politicians only to be ignored. Not even denials were sent back, just complete nothingness. Appointments were never missed and prescribed medications were never abused. None of these behaviors were on the list of manic symptoms. His ability to control the intense impulses he was experiencing once again made him appear healthier to us than he really was. As if that wasn't enough, he had enrolled himself in Certified Peer Support Specialist

145

(CPS) training. He drove himself two hours away to stay at a motel for a week instead of going to the beach with his family ... to celebrate his 30th birthday. The second week of his training, he stayed with another student, who lived locally, that he had met during the training. He spent all of the money he had left in his bank account. She and her husband offered to put him up for the second week to help him save what he had left.

He was never able to get his insurance back in time to help him pay for his ECT treatments. He had to pay out of his savings, an account that no longer existed. Between wedding rings, down payments, mortgages (yes, he was a homeowner at one point) and medical bills, all of the money he had saved was gone. There were no new clothes or fancy dining experiences. He traded in his dream car for an older used vehicle with a substantially smaller monthly payment. This old car had duct tape on it and a garbage bag driver-side window which had become stuck in the down position. He did not spend frivolously, but he still found himself broke; living with his parents. Tending to their home every summer while they went to their beach house, pretending that the work he did for them was equal to the monthly payment he received from them.

He was determined to change his story, no matter what sacrifices he had to make. He quit smoking marijuana completely and devoted his life to this two week course. Not all of his choices were sound, but his determination remained at the forefront of his consciousness. He was not satisfied with his narrative and still, at 30 years old, refused to give up the hope that he was meant to be more.

He was a natural in the training. The only true requirement at the time to be a CPS was to be in recovery from a mental health crisis. The movement was essentially to create professionals in the field who were actually allowed to say: "I know how that feels, kind of." It was the responsibility of the Peer Specialist to be an expert at not being an expert. This was something I did not practice when we first met all those years ago, but I soon became part of the movement too. He became a nurse, in part, because he wanted to do what I was doing. I became a Peer Specialist for the same reason; to be more like him.

He drove home after the first week of training to celebrate his 30th birthday. Not many of his friends showed up. Certainly not as many as had said they would. This was becoming another recurring theme in his life. I remember him saying how he felt as if he was always there for others, but often felt neglected when seeking reciprocity. His mother always tried to persuade him to stop expecting such returns. Intellectually, he was aware of what she was trying to say; emotionally, however, he continued to feel hurt.

Upon returning to his training and staying with one of his classmates and her family, he was able to save some money, which was quickly depleting. Life itself was expensive between car and phone payments, gas, cigarettes, etc. He had not frivolously spent his remaining money, but that didn't mean it wasn't deteriorating. He completed his training with ease, often being taught to practice behaviors he had already tried to implement while nursing. By earning this certification, he felt he would be able to be more open with his care of those suffering. No longer would he have to hide who he was or what he had lived through. It would soon be his professional duty to share his life story, when appropriate, as well as devote more of his time to listening to others going through similar struggles. Although money remained a concern very close to the forefront of his mind, he was now motivated and seeking employment within the mental health field once again.

Chapter 13: Recovery-Focused Care

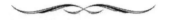

The light was finally peeking through the darkness that was his existence. With a glowing letter of recommendation in one hand, and an impressive resume in the other (both in the mental health field and, now, in the art world as well), he walked into the same hospital in which he received the majority of his mental health care as a teenager and young adult, this time for an interview. The comeback story was impossible to ignore. He breezed through the interviews with a confidence he had not experienced for quite a long time and awaited a phone call.

This is not to say that he had his life under control. Instead, it was as if he had figured out enough of what he was experiencing to control it, with leftover energy to expend professionally. He was charismatic, intelligent, and driven. He was also disillusioned, presenting a front of self-control and awareness that sounded even better when he spoke of it. It required a much keener eye to recognize the continued existence of symptoms. One in which even the professionals he received help from couldn't recognize early on. He found himself closer than ever to being "himself" again, all while remaining in unhealthy relationships with others that had him questioning his core morals and values.

It was as if he was able to convince himself, and others, that everything he was doing was okay, while hiding this secret life from anyone he felt he wouldn't be able to convince otherwise. He was no longer using any substances to maintain a balance other than the medications his doctors continued to prescribe.

He received the phone call he was waiting for and soon had a desk in the same office as the therapists that once worked with him when he was a patient. The job was to incorporate the CPS strategies that were successful during the day shift within the evening shift. This had never been done up to this point at this facility, and therefore his payments came by way of a two year grant. He was to tackle this project with another who was hired alongside him and the full time peer specialist who worked during the day. Within the first six months, he was using his music and computer skills to create presentations that were shared with patients and professionals alike. He even had the opportunity to speak to all of the physicians on staff about medications within the unit!

This is not to say that difficulties didn't arise as well. His partner had already quit, having a mental health crisis due to the stress that this new position, and all of its ambiguities, had created. He was experiencing the same strain, but was unwilling to tap out yet.

Months went by, with empty promises of hiring another to help him with this load he was bearing. Soon, he was offered a charge nurse position on the unit he was doing his work on. He turned it down, remembering all of the times he tackled too much too quickly in the past.

He was determined to avoid another repeat of the broken record that was his life. This time was going to be different. Instead, he took on the project as a solo full-time employee.

The presentations continued. He became the chair of the Relationship-Based Care Committee. With stars in his eyes, he took to the new responsibilities with an intense strategic approach that he was sure would succeed, until he realized he was more of a mascot than anything else. During the monthly meetings with administration and others within the committee he realized that no one was looking to improve. Instead, the higher ups would just tell him that the concerns he was observing were not concerns at all. "How would they know?" he thought early on. "They never leave their offices."

Month after month, he bottled up his frustration until he soon found himself unable to keep these questions to himself, challenging those looking on from afar. Day after day, he remained on the front line, carefully choosing which issues to address out loud to his bosses. Ultimately, it was a losing effort. As those around him encouraged him to fight on behind closed doors, they hid their heads in the sand anytime he tried to advocate to audiences that could actually help implement the necessary changes. He soon felt as if he was drowning once again. However, he had gotten even better at treading water, able to spend more time under intense circumstance.

He decided to try and advocate with assertion, a skill he was taught throughout his time as a patient. Regardless of what facility he found himself in, assertiveness training was part of the therapy. In his youth, he was passive aggressive. In his weakest of states of depression, he was passive. The idea of assertion was as foreign to him as it was imperative. During the manic symptoms he was now experiencing, he found himself ready to fight, appropriately (or so he thought). It was time for him to fight and use everything he had learned to this point to hang on and verbalize his needs. He attempted to explain in writing the current state of affairs regarding this "experiment" he was heading. Here is what he wrote to his superiors:

Evening Shift Peer Specialist Review After 18 Months

I recently attended a webinar with the Crisis Manager on Peers working in crisis as well as the role of a peer specialist in general and how to get the most out of the position. This webinar made me realize a number of different factors necessary for the health of a CPS, as well as the ability to provide high level care and avoid burnout. Throughout my employment, I have been told to "create" this position due to the fact that it had never really existed beyond day shift. I have adapted to multiple variations in scheduling and done my best to also adapt to more than one hardship. I have worked diligently trying to decipher what an "Evening Shift Peer Specialist" is expected to do. Topics I have assessed throughout this process include:

- Difference between day shift and evening
- Role of specific position on evening shift (including necessity of position within these hours)
- Amount of support
- Health of peer specialist on shift

- Overall utilization of my specific skill set

What I have learned is that I have slowly become more of a mental health worker than a CPS. Due to the amount of time spent with consumers and the smaller number of staff in the evenings, I have been the first responder to multiple falls, agitated and aggressive patients, and even consumers who have been lying in their own excrement. Because I am already with the consumers, I am often forced to either engage in the situations that I am told are not my responsibility or leave the situation and look for staff that is already busy with the continued admissions and medication administrations, etc. I have had a very difficult time leaving someone on the ground who has fallen or leaving an unsafe individual with defenseless consumers and, by my own fault I suppose, have put myself in harm's way and overstepped my job description often out of what I believed to be necessity in the moment. One statement that resonated with me during the webinar was:

"You cannot just place a CPS somewhere because it is good to have one. This often leads to compassion fatigue and leads to burnout or even relapses of illness." - Leah Harris, Montana's Peer Network

I understand that I have appeared to be successful in my endeavors as of this time but I am now saying that the shift is not a healthy placement for me.

My main rationale for the previous statement is the idea of support, which was also discussed in the webinar. As a member of the therapy team, I have never been able to attend a therapy staff meeting due to my schedule. I am not invited to the staff meetings involving the people I work with due to the fact that I am not part of that team either. I have no opportunity to interact with doctors, therapists, or social workers, nor be a part in any way of the treatment for each consumer. This is all due to the fact that all of this happens on day shift before I clock in. These interactions are all highly important according to Heather Rae and Paul Lion of Common Grounds stating that "the peer specialist must remain an integral part of the treatment of peers and that their knowledge is as important as anyone's in care." I was a charge nurse on a psychiatric unit as well as a psychiatric coordinator for over 100 consumers. I have a lot to offer based on my history as well as my ability to learn the consumers. I am qualified to do more and I am asking for the opportunity. Other ways of support mentioned included:

- Clinical supervision
- Weekly coaching
- Flexible work scheduling and adequate vacation time

It has been very difficult for me to receive any of this due to the fact that my team is on their way out when I am starting my shift. I am in no way wanting to complain and I am in no way ready to give up. But I am going to protect my health so I can remain employed and be an asset to your company. In order to do this I must advocate to become more involved and also be surrounded by more support so that I do not need to continue re-traumatizing myself with verbally aggressive consumers or medical emergencies in which I am the first responder just based on doing my job as asked. NONE OF THIS IS THE FAULT OF THE OTHER EMPLOYEES on the shift; it is the reality of having a position such as mine in the wrong time slot. I believe that a time change will be helpful also in regard to the new position of RBC chair and RELATE trainer. With the other CPS also working, I will have time to work and implement the different modalities we come up with. My peer has been doing so many groups during the day, my workload continues to increase to a point in which it is becoming more and more difficult to do anything but try and catch up. I am suggesting a discussion of the idea of either:

- A split shift such as 1200-2030 or 1000-1830
- Two CPS working on the day shift

Either of these will allow more attention to be paid to the higher acuity wing as well. Because the acute unit has a faster turnover and the main goal is to meet new admits, having two peers will open up more quality time to be given to the higher acuity consumers.

I appreciate your time in reading this, and hope it makes enough sense that we can set up a time to discuss further whether or not this is a possibility. Thank you.

He continued to fight. He continued to advocate. Again, he found himself crying on his way to work and on his way home. Sometimes, during the more intense pleas, he was even seen with tears in his eyes during meetings and appointments. It was clear in the responses he was receiving from the consumers that he was in the right place, but was he in the right mind? He was hanging out with people 10 years or more younger than him, professional during his shifts and then sophomoric in his free time. The medications were continuing to change. He stuck to the regimens, never abusing or discontinuing anything the doctors were throwing his way, but observing him socially showed that he was rebelling in his own way. Not even he was able to see it yet.

Job? Check.

Insurance? Check.

Self-control?

SELF-CONTROL?

Unfortunately, that box could not be checked yet. Those who knew him better may have seen the signs but he was so clever with his words that he was able to convince them otherwise. Manipulation remained a tool he used during survival mode. As a teenager he used it to hurt others. As a young adult he used it to convince them he was okay. He even began to fall for his own gift of gab.

"Don't believe in your own magic."

A phrase he had heard from his father as he continued to rise through the ranks. The music was pumping his knowledge and message across creatively. His career was allowing him to spread his word professionally. He was never closer to his two paths intersecting, allowing for him to begin fulfilling what he believed was his destiny. He was driving too fast with no brakes. Instead of pulling over and fixing what he knew was broken, he continually challenged himself to perfect recklessness.

He couldn't maintain his pace. He had never made it further, broken. He had never scrapped as hard. He had never remained outside of his comfort zone for such a long period of time. It was as if he returned to his wrestling mentality, refusing to submit, even though all of the signs were there that demise was imminent. He knew how to handle the twists and turns. How to whiz around others, while, for the most part, keeping them at a safe enough distance from the carnage.

There were casualties. Friendships destroyed. Relationships strained. Bonds broken. He had done things, yet again, that went completely against his morals and values, somehow, remaining unscathed himself, but alone. Best friends abandoned him. Religious figures refused to even have conversations with him and companions stopped returning texts until there was nowhere to turn. He was finally met with a situation he was incapable of handling. As if it was his turn to pay for everything he had gotten away with prior to this.

Chapter 14: S.N.A.F.U.

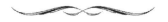

His overuse of social media due to his desire for positive feedback was the last straw. A co-worker saw a picture of him with someone they realized was a former consumer of the facility he currently worked at. Without appropriate fact checking, a colleague assumed he picked her up during her stay at the hospital and went straight to management. It wasn't long before everyone around him believed that he began a relationship with a "patient" to most, but a "peer" to him.

This is not to say that he wasn't aware of the rules nor that he didn't agree with said rules and abide by them. He took his job very seriously, however, his ego remained a vacuous hole that he was now filling with an

163

overconfidence in his athletic frame and recent success. He got called into an office with all of his superiors inside. The situation was explained to him. He immediately broke down but summoned enough guts to ask one simple question: "Did you check my date of hire and her admission and discharge dates?"

He knew full well that they didn't because he was already positive these specific accusations were untrue. The room fell silent. He asked again, more urgently, fearing that his co-workers thought he was some sort of monster. He hadn't met his current companion during her stay at that specific facility. She was actually someone he hadn't even had contact with for quite a long time, years in fact. The perfect storm had arrived yet again, and deep down, he felt he deserved this one more, but not enough to lose everything he had worked for based on a false accusation. The more desperate he felt, the more courageous he became. He began to explain that, due to the fact he hadn't worked during her stay, HIPPA was actually being violated in this disclosure. HIPAA, in short, is basically a confidentiality agreement upheld by all involved in someone's treatment. It was not his business to know whether or not someone he was romantically engaged with had been a patient before he was employed. He pushed back. He gained some leverage and created space, but the end result soon became obvious.

For him, it was a simple request to right this wrong. Send out an email to the entire staff stating that the allegations were false. He did not fear losing his job at this point, he feared working in a hostile environment. Fraternization is not tolerated. It is the responsibility of the professional to abstain. He knew he wasn't completely innocent of the behaviors, but he was innocent of what he was being accused of specifically. Between his own guilt and the paranoia created from whispers and perceived attacks, his house of cards tumbled. He wrote a resignation letter a month after getting his position, that was initially attached to a grant, into the hospital's budget. After achieving the goal he had set, after exceeding all expectations for him and the project, he quit.

As someone who loved chess, he had realized that it would not be many more moves before it was over. His understanding of strategy had saved his integrity before and he felt it time to protect that above all else - retreat in order to avoid surrender. No battle is worth the entire war. Because he hadn't learned to humble himself in time, he was now humiliated. Here is what he wrote:

October 12th, 2015

To Whom it May Concern:

Although it pains me to be writing this document, there are too many inconsistencies in the Certified Peer Support Specialist Position. I have worked incredibly hard in this creation and subsequent addition to the budget and to the team. I have not only offered my services to our consumers but also to our staff through the committees, as well as education, through training and multiple presentations.

I have witnessed in the past months prior to my medical leave, as well as the months following my return, a lack of attention to the suggestions on how to continue to improve the CPS position on the second shift. I have felt an overall lack of respect for the intentions of discussions and also an overall lack of understanding on what the appropriate way to care for those in crisis is. I can no longer continue to expose myself to a unit that is unhealthy for myself, other staff and consumers.

As a nurse, I can no longer expose myself to procedures that are giving our facility a poor reputation on appropriate mental health care. Regardless of what numbers you choose to look at to refute this statement, as a former patient of this facility and as a former charge nurse in the psychiatric field, I am willing to verbalize this without regret.

Nurses must have discretion as far as which admissions are appropriate for their milieu at any given time. We have staff who are willing to work themselves to burnout but administration unwilling to realize the true value of the knowledge and immense skill sets of said staff. I have seen people leave who love this field, I have seen people in charge breakdown during their shift due to a valid inability to maintain a healthy milieu, and I have seen others lose the desire to care for those who are ill, a desire that drew them to this field from the day they applied. I personally have experienced a level of illness that I had not experienced prior to working that specific shift full time. Either our staff are all incompetent or changes must be considered to improve this decline.

The decline has caused those who have always sought help from this facility to go to our competitors, if business must be your main concern. It has caused consumers who admitted the need for help to leave early just to be away from our inpatient unit due to fear, frustration, or lack of continuity of care with staff, doctors, and even policies. The decline has caused consumers to file complaints of incompetency about completely competent staff who have been set up by a faulty system that appears to be unchangeable. The consumers are not wrong about their complaints, the staff are not incompetent, the policies and procedures require a reevaluation. If we want to consider ourselves a Recovery Focused Facility we must first learn what recovery means. The only way to learn that is to actually listen to the suggestions of those on our front lines (staff), and those who are seeking ours services (consumers). Until then, we will use the word "recovery" like any other word, thrown around at our convenience for the sake of creating a guise, an identity that does not represent what we actually offer.

Personally, I have credited part of my recovery to this hospital, and the rest to my determination to never give up. I now find my recovery in severe jeopardy, and my mental health quickly deteriorating. I have been hired to model what a person in recovery is as a Certified Peer Specialist. It saddens me to have to role model that, at this point, by removing myself from employment here, at a mental health facility. I consider exposing myself to the continued lack of conviction as far as how we run our unit now a trigger, one in which I have tried to advocate against for some time now. I have fought and discussed factual information in order to improve one singular position, but the truth is, I have watched people in multiple disciplines breakdown by no fault of their own. I cannot continue to hate the field in which I worked far too hard to excel in. I will not allow any job to be the reason that I once again find myself in crisis. I hope through my own advocacy, your facility will continue to discuss moving forward with your Recovery Movement here, but I can no longer remain a part of this team. I appreciate all of the compassion, support, and hard work of the staff. This hospital will always be the hospital I seek my care from, and I will remain a consumer following my removal from employment.

I appreciate the opportunity and will always be grateful for the care received here. ~ end of letter.

Multiple copies were made and all were signed by his hand. After distributing his letter of resignation, he stopped to talk to one of the social workers about disability benefits. He felt he was unable to avoid situations such as this. No matter where he went, or how hard he worked, he ended up humiliated and seen in a poor regard. This was the beginning of when the line between mentally ill and insane was tiptoed. Luckily, he was smart enough to cushion his descent as much as possible by proactively preparing to receive medical assistance. He knew that he needed some type of insurance to continue receiving treatment. It was these types of choices that we missed from afar, too often only seeing the behaviors that frightened us. This was a clear sign that he was still trying. He required treatment and found a way to continue to pursue health. With this insurance, he made his way into a more intensive outpatient setting. He saw his therapist once a week and remained diligent with his medications. Even in this process, calamity arose.

His previous employer made a documentation error and his insurance was discontinued without him knowing. The insurance provider was under the impression that he was working 40 hours a week, which was far too much income to receive assistance. Once again, money, which he no longer had, was trickling out of his account. By no fault of his own, he was paying full bill for his treatment necessities.

No one, not even I, knew how little he cared about his life. He began to focus more on his music yet again, as he often does when the rest of the world stops making sense. In the last ditch efforts of a dying man, he dedicated himself to the idea that he could do something creative enough to find employment; music, acting, digital art. He spent hours upon hours of his day trying to establish himself creatively. In the meantime, he stocked shelves at a grocery store and moved heavy objects at an antique warehouse; jobs that didn't even last a month for him. He stopped getting paid to help coach wrestling and soon convinced himself he wasn't being appreciated for the work he was doing; a recurring theme, but was it valid?

Food cannot be put on the table as a glorified volunteer. He loved everything he was a part of, but he was no closer to his own independence. It wasn't long before he felt like a joke and believed he was seen the same by those around him. He had survived another crash, but shock was ensuing. I was grateful that he called me the night he checked himself into the hospital that was also his previous place of employment - ballsy. Like many in his life at this time, I was busy with my own existence. I hadn't met with him in years, and assumed, based on our other interactions, that he was succeeding. He didn't need me, there was no way this phone call was due to a crisis. Unfortunately for all of us, it was. No voicemail was left that night. Instead, a voicemail came the following morning from a hospital staff member at the one facility he hadn't yet worked at. He was running.

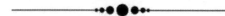

Chapter 15: Different Patient, Same Treatment

The nurse said he checked into the local ER the previous night with a blood pressure close to 220/110 or something absurd like that. Although he has little recollection as to why, even to this day, she explained that he required one to one supervision while in the care of the emergency room staff. There was no bodily injury sustained. He hadn't hurt himself this time. The nurse also stated that he denied having any suicidal ideation. He didn't want to die, he had worked far too hard to quit. It was a desperate attempt to save the ship that had already sunk, again. Yet another recurring theme it seemed. He got checked into a facility about an hour away early the next morning and was placed on suicide watch.

This meant that he couldn't even use the restroom without someone watching him, even though he denied suicidality. I wish I could have been there to help him. I believed that he wasn't suicidal. There was no need to place him on such observations, he was just reaching out for help.

We talked briefly later that day about his current situation. I felt terrible about missing his phone call. I tried my best to keep my selfish guilt out of the conversation, but it didn't stop me from apologizing more than listening. We discussed the idea of him signing a 72 hour notice due to the fact he had voluntarily checked himself in. A 72 hour notice basically means that the staff has 72 hours to prove a necessity for treatment or he is free to leave against medical advice (AMA). This, unfortunately, turned out to make things even worse than they already were.

The doctor who was treating him, a doctor who had never worked with him throughout his almost 20 years of treatment, was now in charge of his future. The choice between rescinding the notice or becoming an involuntary admission was laid before him. In spite of his intense beliefs about this unfair and unprofessional proposition, he chose responsibly and rescinded his request. The following days of treatment were rampant with overmedication and he found himself in the situation he had seen so often as a professional. They weren't listening to him. Those that did, believed him. They did not fight for him though, instead, they tried to teach him how to handle the stress. Those that didn't listen just watched. Decisions in the present were made on his past behaviors and actions during hospitalization, as if that was an appropriate determination of his well-being. He was begging for help, speaking with clear and honest communication all while in a fatal tail spin.

Who wouldn't show symptoms of depression? The situation was depressing.

Who wouldn't show symptoms of panic? The situation was life or death to him.

Which part of his behaviors were concerning, his accurate depiction of what he needed or his unbridled determination to find peace? He loved to try and explain situations to us through comparisons, and drowning appeared to be something people gave more gravity to in the past.

"Imagine drowning and having everyone who loves you standing around shouting 'swim.' If I could swim, I wouldn't be drowning. I wouldn't be screaming for help. You see me treading and think I'm fine, but I'm not. I'm trapped. I'm stuck. I'm just surviving."

Images such as this one made so much sense, and I knew which part of that story I was. I was one of the people standing on the side of the pool shouting "Swim!" I had seen him "swim" before. In my mind, because I knew he could before, I assumed he could now. I disregarded his cries for help under the belief that I knew better. There was nothing more he could have done. Asking for help was a last resort for him when it came to his recovery, mainly to avoid the frustration of others' inability to comprehend his torment. He also felt that he was still keeping them out of his blast radius. It was his to figure out, and the older he got, the more he realized this.

Unfortunately, we didn't realize that he was aware of this, and ultimately continued to fling any and all advice his way, only weighing him down more. You cannot listen while you are talking, and advising is talking. He was no longer in denial, we were. We didn't give him the credit of understanding the condition that he had to live with. Because we, as a society, still understand mental health minimally, we make our own assumptions and deductions about the validity of a "patient's" statement.

How could someone in a crisis speak intelligently? If he knew what was best for himself, he wouldn't be here to begin with, right? I am not here to say that everyone who speaks with clarity during such situations should be given full attention, but what if some people should be? Do ill people not deserve to be a part of their care?

He always believed recovery was a shared goal between him and his supporters. He couldn't understand why anyone, familial or professional, thought they wanted his health more than he did. He lived with this hell everyday of his life for over half of it. He would ask why people were more scared than he was when he was the one living in it. I couldn't answer any of his questions, neither could the staff. Neither could the doctor. However, they chose their hypotheses over his statements. They implemented a treatment plan based on their interpretation of him and did not care for any of his input. "I give up" was the last thing he said to me on the phone. I didn't want to believe him, but I knew he meant it in some form or fashion.

He started establishing social relationships with others under the care of the facility, something he used to refuse to do. He tried to be cool to fit in with the popular crowd and just started putting on a mask that others wanted to see. He acted selfishly and even raised his voice in a group therapy session. He challenged staff and spoke intensely, almost appropriately attacking all around him with his wit. His "why not" mentality was obvious and almost intentional. He was making a statement, becoming what everybody was telling him he already was. The most ironic part of this time period was the fact that when he acted in such ways we told him "wasn't acting like himself." Hmmm, we are telling him he is mentally ill, but when he behaves outside of a certain expectation he is not being himself. It was mixed message number 4,506.

He even set himself up for more self-loathing when a relationship with one of his peers in the hospital immediately imploded following his discharge. His sister was having marital issues and soon it was decided that the two of them switch places because his relationships at home were becoming strained as well. He needed to be somewhere else, and so did his sister. She took his room at their parent's house and he went to live with his brother-in-law, someone he considered more family than a friend.

He had two brothers-in-law that he loved and lost. It was much easier for him to interact with people who weren't part of his immediate family. They appreciated him more, or at least said more compliments out loud to him. They agreed with his rants about the family's weaknesses. He established healthy relationships with older male role models, something he had difficulty doing with his twin brother and father. It was not because they weren't good role models, it was because he believed

179

they never truly understood him. For most of his life, he considered them both to be the catalysts for his treacherous existence. It was always his brother or his father that he would blame internally. He used to tell me that he didn't think they truly understood how important they were to him, or how much he paid attention to their words and actions.

He experienced a great deal of conflict following his inability to sever ties with his brothers-in-law who ultimately weren't able to remain "part of the family" following divorce. But they meant a great deal to him and he fought to maintain relationships with them. At this time, he wanted to be somewhere where he felt more appreciated, and he believed living with his brother-in-law would be a possible quick fix. However, it truly is impossible to run from a lack of appreciation for self, at least it was for him. He used to always say, "Denial is a comfort I am unable to experience."

Posts and pictures flooded his social media stream. He had actually begun to perfect his makeshift digital artwork. He even found himself advertising for the wrestling club he coached at again and soon for a local energy drink. He interviewed with upstart companies and convinced himself there was money to be made. Deep down he felt like he was whoring himself out and selling himself to the cheapest bidder, unless he was doing it for free, which he was also willing to do for exposure at any time. He got to meet his idol, Olympic Gold Medalist Kurt Angle, during this process, and it was the first time he realized that we are all just human beings. There was nothing special about the way his idol looked or spoke. What was special about his idol was the man's work ethic and willingness to push himself harder than anyone around him. He started to realize that the only thing that separates us as human beings is how we act and the choices we make and on this day he decided to live differently. The new strategy was being put in place and his chess board was stacked with the appropriate pieces to attack. He got a gig in a documentary about stigma, but as an actor, not an expert.

Not someone who has experienced it.

Not a mental health professional.

An actor.

He even found himself auditioning with a local youth director to create a musical that educated youth on mental health through entertainment. With a Bluetooth speaker in an empty dance studio, he rapped and sang an original song as a way to showcase his ability and intention. The project was given the green light, and based on the credentials of the person who he was validated by, he believed he was close to achieving his dream.

Chapter 16: Lost

He attended car washes with the kids of the youth group, went on bus trips to New York City, had meetings to discuss moving the project forward, including what his creative needs were, and even learned the "Thriller" dance for a parade.

Marketing was discussed as well as merchandise. A team was put together to make this creation a reality, and he even received a notebook and a wireless printer to do his part, which he did. He wrote and wrote and wrote. He described the characters of his show and what their interactions would be like with each of the other individual characters. The script and score were littered with creative representations of concepts he believed

183

were important for youth to understand during years he considered were emotionally formative.

He brought copies of his initial workups as well as an itinerary to his first meeting with his team. During his second meeting he began asking for feedback and no one had read what he wrote. He was alone at the beginning of the third meeting. He began attending meetings that discussed new projects that had nothing to do with him. The realization was swift and abrupt for him. This was clearly more important to him than the people he thought he was doing it with.

A team was all he needed; people who excelled where he lacked. He was always so willing to compliment and encourage, but he was also crushed when it wasn't returned. He once told me it was hard to create a team of artists. Everyone wants to be the star.

The concept of shared credit is not considered by an insecure ego, and neither is the concept of shared blame. It is a society where success yields a "look what I did" and failure yields a "look what you did."

The people behind the camera, at times, want to be in front of it and are not emotionally intelligent enough to realize that all parts are equally important. He was never trying to be better than anyone, just trying to do his part. He always openly spoke of what he couldn't do, something that many of his peers refused to share.

This type of information is incredibly important in forming a team. Inaccurate self-assessments leave a team disorganized and incompetent. This is not to say that people are not versatile, instead, to say that some people excel in areas that others are just good at. That same person who excels in one area, may be completely incapable in another. If expectations fall on someone to do what they are incapable of doing, the foundation crumbles. That is why he felt communication was so important. He didn't care if you couldn't, but he did care if the team suffered because you said you could, or worse, that you would, and didn't. The idea of "oops" was another convenience he felt he wasn't allowed to rely on.

None of his mistakes were allowed to slide. It was drilled into his head at a very young age when he didn't do his best or completely messed up that he could do better. He soon was as strict on himself as others were around him. His life was filled with malfunctions that he devoted energy towards in order to strengthen his deficiencies, and he was the mentally ill one! It was his understanding that behaviors such as the one previously described were what "normal", healthy, people do. How is it that all of the "normal" people around him were not held to the same expectations? He could not escape the microscope, and he soon realized he was no longer to remain under it. He also realized he was unable to continue to sustain his current life's path.

Weekly therapist meetings and sporadic intensive outpatient visits gave him enough clarity to realize how quickly he was going down. Against everything he believed in, he applied for disability out of necessity. A process he was aware was as arduous as it was time-consuming. It was a process that tested everything he had left, especially his belief in himself and his patience. It was always his intention to avoid this designation. He truly believed there was a place for him in this world but fatigue trumped ambition. As his brain continued to fill with emptiness, there was one remaining sentiment: do whatever it takes to survive.

He joined a study on diet and mood regulation as a test subject. He was required to eat mostly seafood, the one food he hasn't been able to consume since he was a child. Nevertheless, he did it, for over half a year before ultimately proving too unhealthy to even be responsible for his meals. The realization that none of his other pursuits were going to help him regain his adulthood was one he had tried insatiably to avoid. He was doing digital advertisements for different young businesses. He was not being paid for it.

He was coaching wrestling. He was not being paid for it.

He was writing a musical and interacting with youth at least twice a week, but not being paid for it.

He prepared and presented a wellness program on an adolescent psychiatric unit, the same unit he was once in charge of before.

He even found himself at the state capital building to see the debut of the video he was in about stigma.

He also received accolades for his skill and thanks for what he was trying to do, but he ultimately failed.

He remained open to constructive criticism and immune to unnecessary negativity. In his mind, every opportunity to show his worth could be the one that resulted in employment. With more anxiety within him than ever before in his life, he continued to show up, only to be denied repeatedly. He half-heartedly tried to build foundations, instead building more and more resentment towards those watching from their comfort zones as his spiral downward continued.

The people getting paid daily were requesting his services and offering him nothing but exposure. I remember how much he wrestled with guilt over whether or not it was "right" to ask for money when he ultimately just wanted to help others. This was often followed with frustrations over the current status of his disability request, such as the denial of his disability by Social Security and the paperwork involved with the appeal.

Envelope after envelope showed up at his home with impossible deadlines and threats of discontinuation. He was asked constantly to recall his past, one which he was unable to recollect clearly due to the numerous ECT treatments. It took almost two years before he ultimately was asked to appear before a judge and a panel of "experts," ready to determine whether or not he was "sick enough" for aid.

Unfortunately, that time span saw his decomposition near its completion. Relationships all but lost, and those that remained were being stretched beyond repair. He spent the majority of his time in a bed. Over a year of his life spent waiting and panicking, never leaving his room for anything other than physiological needs. His hygiene dissipated with his care for life. He had put everything he had into the idea that his musical would help him out of the pit he was in, only to realize he depended on a team that he didn't truly know. This was a characteristic of his weakened state. He knew all too well the importance and necessity of others. It was also very clear to him that he had limitations, so he clung onto anyone who offered to help. Not everyone chooses their words as meticulously as he now did. Empty promises and complete dismissals had never hurt him more than they did now. Everyone claimed that they were too busy to even respond to communication attempts.

Busy has become one of our greatest deterrents of growth. It is currently a socially acceptable way to avoid leaving our comfort zones. One of those comfort zones we currently reside in is the one where the word "no" seems worse than completely ignoring someone. I did it to him the night he went into the emergency room. I thought it would be better to ignore him than tell him I couldn't talk. I convinced myself I was busy, as if I couldn't FIND time, but the truth is I just chose not to MAKE time. It has never been more acceptable to be lazy than it is in this day and age. We are convinced, because of what we have been taught, that financially driven labor is the only necessary form of work. It is yet another delusion that we live under.

This idea that your work is the reason for your lack of socialization is a childish excuse.

What we do with our time each day is a choice. How egocentric must I have been to believe that I had less time than he did? He was staving off a complete shutdown, running from darkness into darkness. We see so many people succumb to such madness, and yet, as we watched him fight, we asked him to do more or made him operate on our schedules. After all, we were the ones getting paid.

What we were doing must have been more important …

more stressful …

… more necessary?

His life looked easier, so it must have been, right?

He complained less but resented more. His thought processes were long and wordy but his voice was silent. He conserved all of his efforts towards those he believed were still invested in his journey. Those who hadn't given up on him. Those who listened. They were few and far between. Me, his therapist, his mother, his sister, his girlfriend, and his nieces and nephews.

It was an honor to have earned his trust, but the cost was apparent. The restraint he practiced around those outside of his circle was not practiced in more intimate settings. His anger and frustration had peaked, but so had his self control. He was quietly imploding. His intelligence remained but his refusal to speak was one of many clear signs that his fire was dim. During a single instance, he reached out to me, and I pulled away. His words described disaster while his tone reflected desperation. His heart didn't want to fight anymore and his body couldn't. Actions such as mine only proved to him more that he was right about his choice to isolate.

January 6th, 2017

Consumer is a 34 year old Caucasian male. Denies SI/HI. No SIB verbalized or assessed. Remains on mood stabilizers and anti-anxiety medication, as well as a newly prescribed antipsychotic. Admits regulated usage of marijuana as well. Denies regular usage of alcohol, although admits to sporadic binges. Consumed alcohol less than four times in the past year. Smokes one pack of cigarettes every two days. Observed as clean with flat affect, tearful at times. Continues to verbalize a disdain for his life, but reiterates the lack of suicidal ideation. Continues

192

to discuss frustrations with relationship dynamics, continued unemployment, and lack of relief from medications. Discussed possibility of Electroconvulsive Therapy, a treatment that was previously successful. Consumer discussed in detail reasons for reluctance and fear associated with this treatment. Ultimately, consumer agreed with decision. Gave consumer details on how to set up appointment following a referral from his current physician. Spoke of significant other. Discussed feelings of guilt due to lack of emotional availability and "unwillingness to leave my path for anyone." Consumer verbalized that he would remain safe during this process and we discussed the appropriate plans of action in case of crisis prior to consumer departing under own accord.

Louis Bianco RN, CPS - end of visit note.

Sure enough, after two decades of chaos, he found himself in the ECT suite, preparing, yet again, for another series of shock treatments. I understand that this terminology may not seem medically appropriate, but that is what they were. Regardless of how caring and professional the staff was, and, according to him, this staff was as good as any, the reality of the situation scared him. He knew that short term memory loss was looming and he was still clearing the fog in his brain from the previous treatment. He believed in his heart that the first trial had more benefit than detriment. As with many psychiatric treatments, the side effects take shape much sooner than the therapeutic ones.

His life was filled with risk and reward choices that were imperative to his future. Nothing was guaranteed other than the inevitability of his demise if nothing was attempted. He used to hate the idea that people thought he was unable to do things he didn't "want" to. He was currently fighting for disability with electrodes glued to his head. He failed publicly an uncountable amount of times because of his refusal to stop trying. These are situations that no one would choose, but his calling cared little of his preference.

Preference is a convenience. Convenience is a luxury. It was these types of thought processes he needed to insert within his mind in order to do what was necessary long term. He received six treatments that February and March, being driven home mostly by his girlfriend and parents. He was not allowed to drive during this period of time, but he hadn't been driving much prior. No more socializations and parties. No more social media. He began denying himself the comfort of immediate gratification.

Once again, he was in front of his world, vulnerable and broken, but insistent that he knew what he was doing. No more masks. There was that so-called strategy again! His strategies matured as his ego deteriorated. This was not to say that he didn't care about what he needed, I believe he cared more about himself than ever. No, this only meant that he became willing to do whatever was necessary, regardless of perception or opinion. It has always been a trigger of his to be characterized inaccurately in his opinion, but he had little time to worry about such things. He had little time to worry about anything other than the current emergency he found himself in and whatever was needed to begin the long climb upward. His understanding of weakness and strength also matured during this process. He realized his toughness, and in doing so, became less confrontational, and feared confrontation less.

Then ... he disappeared.

By his description, he was shutting down or "losing his mind." Interactions became scarce, although he did try to assure those around him that he was okay. I can still hear his explanations on why he was not "crazy" or why he was exhibiting symptoms of exhaustion, not depression. Although I never said it out loud, I would internally dispute that claim. He didn't interact with anyone. He didn't get out of bed. He was surely depressed. All of his relationships began to collapse under immense pressure.

He pushed his girlfriend far enough away that she wouldn't be crushed under the weight that he was carrying. It was often not a distance she was comfortable with and her comfort was important to him. He continued to allow her to be close enough to feel safe while he ultimately felt more and more threatened. But she never stopped getting closer and he always allowed for her to do so, as she did with him. It remained unclear as to how they would coexist, but there was no denying they were meant to remain a part of each others' lives. The time that they had spent together had opened up old wounds within her as well, and he soon found himself needing to be the emotionally responsible partner while barely keeping his own life together.

He loved her, but he didn't care about anything. Constantly scrambling, they found themselves victims of long text messages and three hour phone calls. He would threaten to leave her and she would become fearful of being abandoned. When she became fearful, she would panic and begin making rash decisions even she didn't want to make. It was her panic that then led to his guilt, a guilt that often kept him from saying what he needed to for his own well being. It was as unhealthy emotionally as it could have been, but their dedication and willingness to communicate kept it alive long after shock ensued.

He knew how wonderful she truly was, as he did about so many others in his life. This was the usual source of his disappointment and frustration during periods of times that she acted out of character in his eyes. He was able to see who she would be, but he missed who she was then. It was because of this that she was bombarded with concepts such as self-honesty and reasons for behaviors that had become conditioned within her prior to meeting him. They were concepts she was intelligent enough to understand when calm. Her mind was the most fertile of soils he had ever planted seeds, and soon it became overgrown. It was often clear to him that her mind was moving faster than her processing skills could manage. The dam had broken, a dam that she built and strengthened from the day she was born, out of her own necessities, some similar to his.

He challenged her as he had challenged all those he cared about, but she was able to see his intentions in a much clearer light. He was so used to being dismissed because of his unwavering demand for someone's best, or dismissing others himself. Somehow, in the midst of his hardest crisis ever, she remained. Broken, but functioning ... barely, and together.

The summer months continued as they had for the past five years he had lived at his parent's home. Each summer his parents would go to the beach and he would toil away at putting his pieces together alone. He was responsible for keeping the affairs in order at the home and maintaining the outdoor areas. Simple enough, but at this time in his life, incredibly stressful. He understood that he needed to do these things, and never argued the understanding that it was his responsibility. His arguments stemmed more from the ideas of, "why are you leaving me alone when I am going through all this? How are you depending on me to uphold your home when my life is in ruins?" In hindsight, he stated he was somewhat fortunate that he had responsibilities, believing they got him out of bed during a time when he "felt no other reason to (get out of bed)."

Other than carrying out those routine chores, he otherwise states a complete lack of memory as to his life in this time. It was as if he set his course and then left his fate in the hands of the elements. He told us he was going to shut down, but my goodness, his auto pilot was impressive. He maintained a relationship with someone he loved during a mental checkout. He kept himself and others safe from harm. He began to show us life again the day he decided to rage against the machine for the first time in his life.

He had won his disability appeal and received back pay from the time he originally applied for the assistance, a two year process before concluding. He had no difficulty being completely honest. It was so hard for him to sit in a room and explain his failure to function while he had just finished his musical. Complete character descriptions, relationship dynamics, and songs with lyrics and music. The entire purpose of the musical was to educate others, hopefully youth, on how to navigate the journey he was returning from himself, symbolizations of important concepts for a healthy mind cleverly entertaining with educational material. He was trying to warn everyone around him of the dangers he witnessed in forms of communication that seemed to reach youth. His dedication to message delivery may be the reason he reaches his final destination, but that remains to be seen. Nevertheless, there he was, in front of a judge, crying and submitting ... again. Ultimately he "won," and now with some money in his bank account again, he continued to make decisions he felt were in his best interest.

Chapter 17: Withdrawal

"If I'm wrong about this then you are right, I really am delusional, but let me try. Either I will be right or I will be crazy, but at least we will all get our answer."

This was what he said after we discussed him discontinuing his medications completely. No professional ever wants to hear a mentally ill patient challenge medications. His whole life he was told that such an idea is a sign that the illness still exists. He never challenged the idea of medication, but here he was, 34, heavily medicated, unemployed, and in pain. He checked himself back into the intensive outpatient program he had received so much guidance from. All on his own, he planned an appropriate attack and used the resources provided to him to create a path to health.

He did not have to rush towards anything other than sanity at the moment. Employment was not his most pressing issue currently, life was; and plenty of work was necessary. He began requesting blood work, knowing that some of the physical symptoms he was experiencing were not normal to him. His doctor continued to explain to him why blood work was unnecessary and why his panic was symptomatic of his diagnosed illnesses. So he told his doctor that he was going to quit taking medications and requested a professional titration plan.

"I am not trying to make myself worse, I am trying to get better. This is the only thing we haven't tried yet."

So it happened, under the care of professionals, Monday through Friday from nine to three, he began slowly weaning off medication. Close to 20 years of medication had become part of how his system developed, altering forever the chemistry within his faculties. Slowly, at first, he recognized his body's longing for chemicals that were no longer present. His withdrawal was like moving slowly towards the waterfall, but ultimately, it's still a waterfall and off you will go. Free falling scared him more than anything. There is no control in a free fall other than your level of calm.

His extremities became numb randomly as he shivered in his own sweat. His heart beat out of his shirt to remind him that he had forgotten to exhale. Holding his breath for long periods of time unknowingly was one of the scariest side effects he experienced. He described it to me as being underwater yet again. It was something people could relate to - the way your heart starts to react when it realizes the oxygen is gone.

Some people can stay underwater for long periods of time, perhaps even ignorant to this survival mechanism. Others immediately panic and surface, gasping for air. He was somewhere in the middle, realizing the gravity of what caused the panic response, but not reacting to said panic. He trusted his panic response, but wanted to improve his response to it. Again, as someone who had experienced trauma, his threat detection had long been skewed, going into protective mode sometimes at the hint of danger. This was yet another way he improved his thinking, the transition from fear being a deterrent to a catalyst. The recognition of fear as a challenge that required his highest attention and focus.

"All you can do is survive as long as possible. The calmer you are, the longer you have."

This doesn't mean that he wasn't panicking internally.

It doesn't mean that he didn't crack and seek to be held in the arms of anyone willing to see how hard he was grinding.

It doesn't mean he didn't yell and tantrum about fairness and who's fault his life was. It just meant that, when he came face to face with every fear he ever possessed, he looked it in the eye and refused to budge. His greatest achievement was his greatly improved stress tolerance, and it is probably the reason he remains alive.

It was ugly at times. The fear in his eyes was evident and intense. So many aspects of his journey were ugly, and withdrawal is not a pretty business. However, even while going off benzodiazepines, mood stabilizers, and antipsychotics, he pushed his treatment forward and ultimately scheduled labs with his primary care physician (PCP). He lost control of his emotions during the appointment, crying out to his lifelong doctor, "How did this become my life?"

His doctor did his best to explain different lifestyle changes he could make to reduce his current level of internal agitation. He explained thought processes that may create pain or increase the actual sensation of pain. The doctor listened intently, as always, while he took deep breaths to slow his accelerated system down. The initial results of the blood work came days later, noting results of concern with his blood levels and some liver enzymes. His spleen was enlarged and palpated during initial assessment. His platelets were low. On the exterior, skin was flaking off of his pale face, as his dark sunken eyes appeared black and blue. His hairline receded further and further back at an accelerated rate. He hadn't harmed himself, there just appeared to be bruising underneath his eyes. He even began wearing sunglasses indoors. He was then recommended to get x-rays, head and body scans, and more blood work to figure out what was causing the abnormalities.

HIV and Hepatitis screens began rolling through the order sheet and his panic increased. He knew, intellectually, that this was not the case for him, but kept thinking, "What if?" He did not believe he lived a life that put him at risk for such ailments but he was also aware that he didn't always make the best choices about his physical health. His body was breaking down and he had only been off his medications for a little over a month. It was during this time he arranged a dental visit to have his teeth examined.

Dental hygiene was often neglected during his tougher periods in life. He gave up cigarettes and even his experiments on how to appropriately medicate with marijuana. He rid himself of all chemical dependence and sought to find what was causing his physical decline.

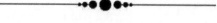

Chapter 18: Still Standing

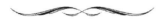

Ultimately, he received a diagnosis. It wasn't HIV. It wasn't hepatitis. Instead, they told him he had idiopathic thrombocytopenia, or low platelets for an unknown reason.

Unknown?

Every specialist he had seen prior to this new diagnosis told him that his prolonged medication use could definitely cause some of the abnormal lab results. They discussed how it was very possible that two decades worth of medicating may have harmed his body, yet the cause was unknown? He was told by medical professionals that he was just exaggerating his experiences and denied follow up lab work. Now he was being told that he actually did have something wrong with him, giving vial after vial of blood at every appointment he attended with a hematologist. These tests and appointments were happening every three months, but his own psychiatrist wouldn't even draw the first blood sample initially. He hasn't gone back on medications and his psychiatrist recently told him he is in remission from his mood disorder.

Now, only a few months since the discontinuation of psychiatric medication, all of the experts he designed his life through are changing their story! Is that even possible? I started thinking more and more about some of his "rants" and realized so many truths about his concerns.

I started putting the pieces together frantically only to come to a conclusion he had figured out years before me. In classic human fashion, his life finally made sense to me. I believe it had made sense to him much earlier, but he realized through disappointment what happens when you try to explain something to a person who believes they know better. In his youth, I believe he tried harder to convince people he was suffering, but in his young adulthood, he became a much more vulnerable person out of necessity. Using everything he learned, he had begun to speak very honestly and clearly about his need for help. In a period of time when no one in his life seemed able to help him, he helped himself once more. He remained on this new found pace he created and understood that he was far from done.

He is now seeing an employment specialist and about to move out of his parent's house. He will be living with the same girlfriend mentioned previously. They have been together for almost two years now. It hasn't even been a year since he received his disability designation. It has only been six months since he stopped medicating himself. We met up recently because I told myself I would no longer allow my own perception of his situation to create any further neglect. I finally learned how to listen to his words. He wasn't being cryptic anymore. He wasn't exaggerating and there were no hidden messages. I know in my heart I never meant to neglect him, but in truth, I never made an effort not to. As he has gotten older, he has chosen to verbalize much more about the way his mind works. At many parts of his journey, he had explained what his needs were. During most of those same instances, I listened, and then explained what I felt he needed more.

Most interventions, then, involved building foundations around what we thought about him, as if we knew better than he did for the rest of his life, no matter how much work he put into his care. He never claimed to be all knowing, but he refused to believe anyone knew him better than he did after decades of internal self exploration. No one in his life had worked harder on self-improvement. Where others were always saved by the excuse of "that's just who I am," he was stuck with the idea that he could always do better. Because he held himself to this standard, as the designated mentally ill person, he held the healthy masses responsible for the same integrity. When we showed our true colors or our own chosen ignorance of our shortcomings, he became frustrated.

Once a month, he speaks to others in similar situations at the same outpatient facility he attended so many times in his life. As a volunteer, he goes to the facility he used to work at, at the request of the therapists within the program, to motivate and encourage. He tells the truth about his experiences and asks that others find the ability to do the same. He doesn't post about it on social media, in fact, he hasn't used that for some time now. He has even deleted some of his more popular music videos because he doesn't believe that he is the same person he portrayed publicly.

His words are still loaded and intense. His communication direct and his eye contact never wavering. He has meant everything he has ever said during serious conversations, and I was finally willing to listen, in our last appointment ever. I was no longer able to refuse my friendship to a person I admired. Although I stopped documenting him, I never stopped listening, and I never will. He has never asked for anything he wasn't willing to give back.

I am a better person now than I was before and he played a role in that.

We still talk in depth about how he became what he is. Is he really disabled because of an inevitable mental illness or was he just a product of a flawed system that is still trying to figure out solutions? He tends to believe both. He believes he has a condition, but if he is ill, who isn't?

Wednesday, April 18th, 2018 @ 1200

Consumer is a 34 year old Caucasian male. Currently denies SI/HI with no SIB assessed. Currently not on any psychiatric medications. Denies alcohol usage, but continues to verbalize usage of marijuana. Admits experiencing certain cognitive discomforts that are alleviated by this, but continues to verbalize fear of law enforcement and frustration that he is "somehow not qualified to receive medical based on diagnosis." He remains determined and willing to do whatever it takes to find some sort of health. He admits to a continued battle with cigarettes but continues to stay present mentally about his usage and remains confident he will discontinue his need to smoke. States that his overall disdain for current life situation is blunted by how he currently regulates himself chemically, often able to continue his efforts forward with its aid. Explains a continued willingness to do whatever is necessary, but refuses to take previously prescribed medications due to continued physical ailment. He described a desire to achieve what he

212

believes is his destiny, even at the cost of long life. Discussed continued volunteering to help those putting their lives back together. Discussed efforts with caseworker and employment agency to begin part time employment. Verbalized fear of trying and failing again but continues to describe a drive that is undeniable. States feeling driven and exhausted simultaneously on a daily basis. Consumer believes he has a message that he must share with others. Consumer continues to write, refining his musical, and even working on a book. "I just need to get this message out. I keep trying to find a method of delivery that will actually be heard. Contrary to popular belief, I don't care how noticed I get. I want to make enough money to allow me to responsibly continue on my path and become a husband and father. I don't care about the clothes I wear or the cars I drive. I have been a psychiatric nurse and a peer specialist, as well as a patient. I have been a rapper. I have acted and spoken publicly. I don't care which way I have to do this, I will do it. I care about others. What they think is very important to me because I am trying to make something for them. I don't want to hear that I shouldn't care about others, as if my desire to fit socially is a weakness. I have a lot to say and I am finally finding my voice. I am going to write a book where I present my life through the eyes of a mental health

213

professional, who is actually me as well. Basically, I am going to write my story as if I were the point person in my own mental health care. I won't tell anyone that both parties are me until the end. I am sure people who know me will recognize very early that it's me, but the story needs to be told."

Humm. I like that idea ...

Louis Bianco RN, CPS — end of visit note.

EPILOGUE

That is right, he and I are one and the same.

I am a 34 year old American male living with his retired parents. I carry the legal designation of disabled. I have shown multiple times an inability to function in society. I am unemployed with an RN and a Peer Specialist Certification. I have to visit a hematologist every three months. My resume is scattered with a plethora of work experience in numerous disciplines, yet it is also riddled with failed attempts of sustained employment. One of the biggest misunderstandings about my case, however, was my discipline and record keeping.

215

I am not here to bury any facility or professional.

In truth, if my life was different in any way, I too would be different. For the most part, it was the guidance and intervention I received from the mental health system that got me this far. However, I also believe that it was the same guidance and intervention that held me back. I hope I can explain more clearly what I mean through writing.

They told me at a very young age that I was experiencing something that was chronic. It was explained to me that this meant I had an illness that I could never rid myself of. They told me which symptoms I had and even explained warning signs that those symptoms were coming. What they didn't understand was how I handled this information. Regardless of why, it was never assumed that I would listen to this information verbatim and make sure to do everything the experts told me to, everything the adults advised.

I am not rebellious by nature. I believed the experts … the adults.

What I failed to recognize in my youth was that everyone was as confused as I was. Some people were even more fearful than I was, and we all know what types of decisions people make during panic. It is a strange mix of intending to help others but ultimately alleviating one's own discomfort. I believe that a large amount of us have a difficult time deciphering between what we do for others and our own personal gain. This has nothing to do with blame. There is nothing wrong with personal gain, other than the unwillingness to admit its necessity. Between parents and teachers informationally unequipped for this situation, professionals somewhat recklessly throwing facts around, and my youthful inability to handle stress appropriately, my life changed forever.

My overall genetic hypersensitivity became a cause for concern. My intense range of emotional responses became proof that I was sick. Having my feelings hurt by words was my fault, even if those words hurt. It was expected of me at a very early age to fix something that, as an adult, I don't even believe is broken. The idea that it was broken was obviously based on observations of behaviors. However, all behavior has meaning, and the first time I truly broke down, it was because of a complete

217

inability to understand what was happening. It was an act of frustration and building rage, and I handled it in an age-appropriate "inappropriate" way. One of the tragedies of this story was the overreaction to the negative, and an underreaction to the positive.

I do believe I exhibited a skill set and intelligence at a very young age that was noteworthy. I knew how to make others laugh and had the same quick wit as my father. The fact that I actually tested as gifted was rarely discussed and I don't even know my IQ to this day. I understand why my mother kept this information from me and I rarely find myself wondering what my IQ is. Who cares?

The only reason I find this information pertinent is because of all the confidence I was not able to derive from this distinction. I always felt, and was treated as if, my best was the same as everyone else's best. I wasn't special. This doesn't mean I wasn't loved or told I was talented. It was just always the immediate safeguard to explain to me how many other people were as talented or even more talented than I was.

Years of keeping my head out of the clouds actually left my head in my hands. I was humbled to the point of believing that I was often lesser than the rest of my family when I was succeeding. When I screwed up, the expectation of knowing better came from every direction. I was always expected to be the bigger person while being told, medically, that I was lesser than. I was the person with the diagnosis, therefore no one else could possibly be at fault for any misunderstanding. As is seen often in traumatic situations, the delegation of power was done hastily, and many people found themselves in roles that didn't flatter their abilities, including me.

I assumed the role of the victim. I believed that the fear around me was as real as it was portrayed by others. I followed the lead of people who, most times, were more scared than I was. Instead of reassuring them to feel calmer, I convinced myself I was not fearful enough. Do not get the misconception that I am saying the person experiencing the crisis should be in charge of steering the ship, but they should be involved. It was my responsibility to learn to communicate with others so that they knew better how to help me. I did not put enough

219

work into my actual role and instead continued to morph into something I wasn't - disabled. My learned dependence led to me doing whatever I was told, and then being frustrated or defeated after inevitable failure. I was being groomed to be something completely opposite of what I was.

Fear is the reason I allowed this to happen, and I meant to say allowed. Consciously or unconsciously, I never made the choice to change my own behavior, specifically my involvement in confrontation. As I stated earlier, I hate confrontation. I avoided it at all costs for the majority of my life and lived an existence of obedience and resentment for my efforts. I didn't speak up because I was afraid of the others around me seeing defiance, often a symptom of multiple mental health diagnoses. But this doesn't mean I couldn't have.

Within my own understanding of how the world worked, as a teenager, I assumed that I knew the end result of standing up for myself. I convinced myself that I knew how each person involved in my care would act. This type of fortune telling is one of the main reasons relationships in modern society are failing. I believe it to be the reason even more mistakes are made. How many times have you heard someone plead innocence to a mistake through explaining what they thought was going to happen. It is not the fault of the universe if you guessed the future wrong and acted, or in my case, didn't act. It is the fault of the person who guesses and guesses wrong. I constantly passed the ball to those who called for it, only to watch them act outside of their abilities and ultimately turn it over.

"They should have done this."

"You shouldn't have done that."

We all seem to believe we know what is going to happen next and plan accordingly to our premonitions instead of acting accordingly to what is happening at any given time. Then we excessively critique it after the fact. Past and future. We operate more and more often within these two times, completely ignoring the present's significance. We all see things differently, I get it. I would hate to insult the quality of anything you like because I would obviously be wrong. You are obviously right all the time, because it's you. Far be it from me to infringe upon your perception of anything.

But what if your perception is only meant for you?

Isn't it possible that, although it's yours, it could be inaccurate?

Couldn't your tolerance for fear affect how you perceive a threat?

Couldn't your life experiences shape how you view danger?

What about your desire to be unique or edgy?

What about your desire to feel part of something or be liked?

Now, imagine that it is your responsibility to treat a mentally-ill child based solely on your perception. Imagine being allowed to mess up under the guise of psychology being an imperfect science. The safety of being in control with no repercussions often leads to impulsive decision-making and a lack of accountability. The phrase "perception is reality" has done more harm

222

than good for our society. I find "your perception is your reality" to be much more accurate. Now insert everyone you interact with and realize that they have their own perceptions as well.

Whose perception is actually reality now?

Is there any common ground that all parties can agree on?

Is there any shared reality within our interactions, or are you immediately all knowing because "perception is reality?"

In many perceptions, we believe we are always the victim or the victor, the lead in their own story, saving the day or being wronged in every interaction they experience; the bravest hero or the most justified villain. Unfortunately, sometimes in life we are just extras. Not everyone is meant to be the star. Not all who are meant to be stars become them. There is a lot that needs to be earned in life, and a lot of work and effort involved in reaching one's full potential. Perception allows us to believe we are more or less at any time, allowing us to keep our egos fed when we don't feel special enough.

Inaccurate perceptions allow us to make poor decisions that could hurt us and those around us. Again, it all goes back to understanding limitation and strength. In team settings, the unwillingness to admit limitations can ultimately sabotage the team's success. I don't want to be on a team with someone who believes they can make every shot. I want to be on a team with a person who gets open where they can make most shots. By sharing a reality, a team can function at a much higher level mentally, making better decisions in each moment to reach an agreed goal. Not everyone who calls for the ball is meant to take the last shot, regardless of what their perception is. In my case, between the perception of others and my own perception of myself, I believed I was sick and acted as such. I joined others perceptions and disregarded my own due to my perception of adult vs. child roles.

The more I earned, however, the more of a role I wanted. As my perception of myself changed, I didn't force others to believe the same, I showed them through my behaviors. If their perceptions of me remained the same, they weren't paying attention. I began paying more and more attention to every little detail about human interaction and behavior. My life was devoted to analyzing myself and I found the greatest results in my growth when I gathered the most data. Soon, I learned how to observe objectively, even within more intimate interactions.

I began learning how to immediately recognize my fault in conflict and admit it. I refused to take complete blame in anything but realized that I had as much, if not more, of a responsibility as any in fixing this. I still didn't believe I broke it, but I understood now that fault had nothing to do with the solution.

I am not who I was. I have lived many lives already in my youth, one of them being egocentric. My perception of normal and concept of worth were dangerously skewed and I spent years of my life meeting selfish needs, sometimes recklessly. I am not innocent in this life nor exempt from the choices I made. There are some people in this world who may hate me, and rightfully so. I have had apologies go unforgiven and for good reason. I will take certain sins to my grave with me and pray for forgiveness every day of my life.

With all of that being said, I still believe I am a good man, and I truly believe in my role on this earth. It is because of this belief that I continue to resurface with my message, always more refined and more controlled with every resurrection.

It is very easy to see a person's true intentions through their behaviors. Like my intentions, for example. Someday, people will look back at my catalogue of work and realize that I have had the same message for my entire life. Sure, I may have tried to communicate it through vehicles that were part of pop culture, but that was just because I felt it needed to be heard by as many ears as possible.

I didn't just keep cursing out of my lyrics for kids. I did it for those older than me. I didn't refuse to curse because I wanted to be different. I did it because I wanted to be heard. I did it so I could use my music in presentations for medical professionals and students alike. I am not a starving artist. This misconception infuriates me. I have a job to do. I learned so much during my hell, most importantly that it didn't need to be this hard. If a map didn't exist before I set sail, it will exist now that I survived the voyage. I didn't only survive, I paid attention to many details and now I just want to share what I learned with others who may be lost.

I have so much to do, yet I can't prevent myself from heading back into the storm every single time I get well enough to do so. The idea that there are so many circling their grave in the darkness relentlessly reminds me that I must share my light. It is not a light that requires a paycheck to remain lit, nor is it a situation in which I have time to negotiate. There are millions of people refusing to give up, treading water. They are exhausted and frustrated, but driven, just like I am. This isn't the type of situation I can just get myself out of and be satisfied. I know how hard my life was and will remain to be because of mistakes that were made. Mistakes that I have spent my life critically thinking about.

I am gifted, the paperwork says so.

I am educated, my nursing license says so.

I am experienced, my medical charts and resume say so.

I am creative and my portfolio says so.

I am everything I claim to be and able to show all of my work as proof, not just my words. I was what I was and I am what I am. Any success I may experience surely wasn't gifted to me, it was earned. I served my time and paid dearly for my lapses of judgement. It is not my fault that I am back still trying, it is a testament to my character. If that is something that makes others uneasy, it is time I ask them to check themselves.

I don't doubt my decision-making any longer. I am no longer questioning my ability to live with what I am. My greatest learning tool has been my listening. There is so much you can learn about someone's illness from them. There is so much they can learn about their own illness from themselves. It is through conversation, not documentation, that such realizations are made, although documentation is extremely necessary.

If one's sole intention is to assess, they are not listening. They are waiting to hear what they feel they need to hear, disregarding any other information. The roles of professional and patient are immediately established and soon the interrogation begins. One person asks, one person answers. There is no discussion. There is no problem-solving, only problem recognition.

Motivating someone to learn more about themselves is much easier when they are allowed to be the teacher. I always felt in some way that I understood a person after meeting them just once, and I also believe that they were able to understand themselves better following our interactions. The best way to do this professionally was for me to make sure my peer controlled the conversations. I deferred control. I didn't forsake any professional responsibilities and remained aware of my role, but I got in the passenger seat. I reiterated what they said. I became a mirror.

At times, I provided thought provoking questions that they then thought about. Because it was a question they never asked, the answer was one in which they had never thought. With each new thought, more and more pathways opened up allowing said person to start filling in more blanks. This cannot happen if I continually tell them what their answers should be. It didn't work for me to be told what I was, especially when I was also being taught to define myself.

The therapist and the psychiatrist don't share many constituencies as far as how they practice, and the psychiatrist usually wins in decision-making. They went to school longer. They are the doctors. I always appreciated the doctors who listened to the staff around them professionally, and the doctors who listened to me as a patient. I did not do well with anyone who thought their paycheck made them better than me. I respected everyone else's intelligence, but not at the sake of having mine insulted.

Based on my story, there was definitely something wrong, and I am grateful for everything I learned now. I can't have any of my life back. I can't undo what was. I have apologized, and exposed myself to more scrutiny than any others in my life could be brave enough to do. I've exposed my indiscretions. I could not run from any of my mistakes and therefore, I didn't. Because I didn't run, I was granted the opportunity to pay for what I did. Because I took that opportunity, I suffered. Because I suffered, I grew. Because I grew, I sought forgiveness. I forgave myself. I admit that some of my bigger mistakes affected many beyond myself but I also admit that I have busted my ass to improve upon my control. I accepted every challenge and I am still standing, fists raised, ready to fight whatever is next.

Stigma exists.

We are becoming more and more educated on symptoms, at least when we see them in others. I am sure to many onlookers, and maybe even professionals, I am delusional. I am hypersensitive and unreliable. My speech is pressured and I care too much about others. I get my feelings hurt when you don't keep your word as an adult. I am idealistic and naive. I am not as important as I believe I am and I am nowhere near as amazing as you are. With my head in the clouds, I am chasing a dream that is impossible. I am a starving artist who wants to be a rapper and perform hip hop. I want to be a star, but I am not special! I am on disability because I am lazy and don't know how to toughen up and do what I have to do. I am weak. I am broken. I am mentally ill, how could I understand relationships or hard work? I don't have a job, how could I know what it means to do something difficult? All of these are possible perceptions, and all of them are false.

Here is the truth about me. If I am delusional, my message is my delusion, but this "delusion" is the reason I keep fighting. It is the reason I try hard all the time. It is the reason I set boundaries and the reason I continue to challenge myself to be better. It is the reason I avoid getting in trouble. It is the reason I deny myself unnecessary urges. My message spurs my work ethic during periods of justified exhaustion. I don't believe that I can do any of this by myself, but I won't stop doing it just because someone's perception is wrong.

I am not going to give up. How many years did I spend keeping others comfortable at the cost of fulfilling my own goals? This lack of fulfillment has kept me humble, and for that I am grateful. However, I will not go back to humiliation. I am too proud. I have worked too hard and for too long. Your perceptions are now yours and yours alone. Think what you must.

What do I think, you ask?

I believe I have information that will help children avoid this hell. I don't think I am the only one who has lived this or will live this someday. I have education and work experience to be taken more seriously by professionals. Education matters. Experience matters. I have both.

I will reach my destination because of preparation, resilience, and courage. When I cross my finish line, a race no one was ever capable of achieving other than me, I will receive what I earned. I will celebrate with those who loved me and believed in me. I will cry and I will pat myself on the back and surely hug those closest to me, and thank them. And, as the dust settles and the initial high fades, I believe I will seek solitude for a moment, filling in my own blanks that have been left open for so long. I will say, "we did it," not "I told you so." I am sure I will feel more satisfied with myself and possibly even look forward to life again.

There are many answers I hope to find after I survive this storm, but I am afraid there is still one I will not be able to answer: Am I disabled?

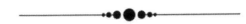

About the Author

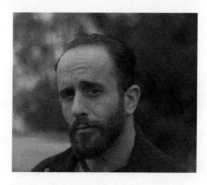

Louis Bianco RN CPS is a 36-year-old native of Central Pennsylvania. Over the past 20 years, he has been a part of the mental health system in PA, as a consumer, a peer specialist, and a psychiatric nurse. He has worked professionally as a Charge Nurse at the Pennsylvania Psychiatric Institute and was able to secure an evening shift Certified Peer Specialist Position into the Budget of Holy Spirit Hospital's inpatient unit through a two-year grant.

Louis has also received treatment for mental illness in this area since the age of 15. He has gone through countless medication regiments, received multiple ECT treatments, and even participated in a dietary study at Hershey Med. Louis has worked at a number of the facilities where he has also received care from. He has devoted his life to the field of mental health and has used his unique perspective to help educate not only those in the mental health field, but also the criminal justice, education, and legal systems as well.

Although currently unemployed and on disability, Louis has continued to advocate for a greater understanding of mental health in the state of Pennsylvania, through close to four years of volunteering as a public speaker and advocate. In 2019 alone, He has spoken at a state conference for health educators about the creation of K-12 curriculums. He has sat on a panel with police officers and caseworkers to discuss mental health to criminal justice majors at West Chester University. He has spoken to over 700 high school sophomores at Cumberland Valley High School's First-ever Wellness Summit. This is the same high school he went to where he first experienced a crisis that had him doing most of his school work in psychiatric facilities! Louis has even had opportunities to speak to politicians and Dickinson Law students preparing to graduate! He continues to find entertaining and inspiring means to deliver vital information on how we can be proactive in the care of our mental and emotional wellness.

Louis continues to do everything within his power and resources to get his message out to the public. Although *Mental Health DisABILITY: Perception vs. Reality* is his first published book, he has dispersed a number of his early curriculums to professionals across the state in multiple fields. There were several obstacles in Louis' way many years ago, and it is his intention to aide in the improvement and unification of all systems involved in the mental wellness of human beings, regardless of age, to help avoid any unnecessary trauma involved in such a difficult journey.

E-mail: LouieJoJo@msn.com

Website: www.reverbnation.com/LouieJoJo

Made in the USA
Columbia, SC
18 November 2021